ABC of
the First Year

Sixth Edition

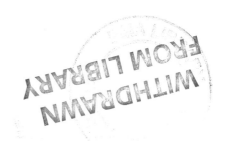

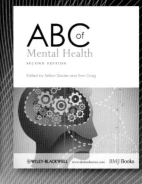
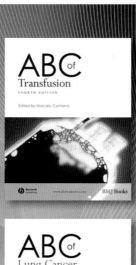
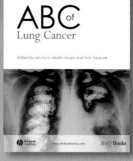
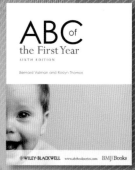
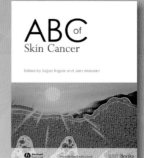
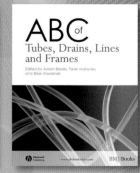

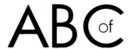

ABC of

the First Year

Sixth Edition

Bernard Valman

Consultant Paediatrician
Northwick Park Hospital
London, UK

Roslyn Thomas

Consultant Paediatrician
Northwick Park Hospital
London, UK

WILEY-BLACKWELL

A John Wiley & Sons, Ltd., Publication

BMJ|Books

This edition first published 2009, © 2009 by B. Valman & R. Thomas
First edition published 1980 by BMJ Books

BMJ Books is an imprint of BMJ Publishing Group Limited, used under licence by Blackwell Publishing which was acquired
by John Wiley & Sons in February 2007. Blackwell's publishing programme has been merged with Wiley's global Scientific,
Technical and Medical business to form Wiley-Blackwell.

Registered office: John Wiley & Sons Ltd, The Atrium, Southern Gate, Chichester, West Sussex, PO19 8SQ, UK

Editorial offices: 9600 Garsington Road, Oxford, OX4 2DQ, UK
                    The Atrium, Southern Gate, Chichester, West Sussex, PO19 8SQ, UK
                    111 River Street, Hoboken, NJ 07030-5774, USA

For details of our global editorial offices, for customer services and for information about how to apply for permission to reuse the
copyright material in this book please see our website at www.wiley.com/wiley-blackwell

Library of Congress Cataloging-in-Publication Data

Valman, H. B. (Hyman Bernard)
ABC of the first year / Bernard Valman, Roslyn Thomas. – 6th ed.
    p. ; cm.
  Includes bibliographical references and index.
  ISBN 978-1-4051-8037-5 (alk. paper)
  1. Infants–Medical care–Handbooks, manuals, etc. 1. Thomas, Roslyn. II. Title.
  [DNLM: 1. Infant, Newborn. 2. Child Development. 3. Infant Care. 4. Infant, Newborn, Diseases. WS 420 V196a 2008]

  RJ48.V28 2008
  618.92′02–dc22
                                                                                              2008006129

A catalogue record for this book is available from the British Library.

Set in 9.25/12 pt Minion by Newgen Imaging Systems Pvt. Ltd, Chennai, India
Printed in Singapore by COS Printers Pte Ltd

1   2009

Contents

Preface to the Sixth Edition

The First Year of Life was the first series of ABC articles commissioned and published weekly by the *British Medical Journal* and later collected and published as a book. The fifth edition was called *ABC of the First Year* to identify it with the ABC series. The ABC series is continuing to tackle new subjects in all branches of medicine and surgery: more than 50 series have been published and 43 books are still in print. The first edition of *The First Year of Life* was printed in black and white and some colour was introduced in the fourth edition. The ABC series of books has been relaunched with a new format and all the illustrations are in colour. Each chapter has been thoroughly revised with considerable changes in several chapters. The latest recommendations of the Department of Health for developmental review have been incorporated and there is a new chart for developmental assessment at any age. The latest clinical guidelines published by the National Institute for Health and Clinical Excellence (NICE) have been reviewed during the preparation of this edition. New sections were added in the last edition on the infant of low birthweight at home, advice on travelling abroad with an infant, and paediatric HIV infection.

The book was written for family doctors, GP vocational trainees, medical students, midwives, and nurses. It has become the standard textbook for several undergraduate and postgraduate courses. The emphasis has been on the practical aspects of management, based on clinical experience, but theory is introduced where it is essential for understanding the basis of management. No previous experience of paediatrics is assumed.

We thank Mary Banks who has been the midwife for several previous editions and Adam Gilbert who has joined her for this edition.

For ease of reading and simplicity a single pronoun has been used for both feminine and masculine subjects; a specific gender is not implied.

Bernard Valman
Roslyn Thomas

Foreword to the First Edition

The care of infants and their mothers has changed rapidly in the past 10 years and it is often difficult to identify those advances that will prove of lasting value to the clinician.

Dr Bernard Valman's articles on the first year of life, published recently in the *BMJ* and collected in book form, aim at providing the clinician in the community and in hospital with generally accepted views on the medical management of infants. The main difference between paediatrics and general medicine is the range of normality, which changes with age. The greatest changes occur in the first year of life. Dr Valman's articles provide an account of normal development during this year, with particular emphasis on its assessment, so that deviations may be easily recognised. These articles have been collected together to provide a practical guide for general practitioners and the many other staff who care for the new born and young infants.

Stephen Lock
Editor, *BMJ* 1980

Acknowledgements

We thank Wiley-Blackwell Publishing for allowing us to adapt liberally material that has appeared in *Practical Management of the Newborn, Accident and Emergency Paediatrics*, and *Paediatric Therapeutics* and use of the two photographs of resuscitating a newborn.

We also thank Susan Thomason, Maire Sullivan, Richard Bowlby, Joanne Fairclough, Brian Pashley, Jeanette McKenzie, Derek De Witt and Ann Shields of the Department of Medical Illustration at Northwick Park Hospital for taking most of the photographs. the remaining photographs were supplied as follows:

Early prenatal diagnosis: ultrasound scans courtesy of Dr H B Meire and Sujata Patel.

Breathing difficulties in the newbourn: micrograph of respiratory distress syndrome courtesy of Dr J Wyatt-Ashmead; apnoea monitor, Graesby.

Some congenital abnormalities: cleft lip, courtesy of Mr R Saunders.

Routine examination of the newborn: cardiac ultrasound, courtesy, of Miss Varrela Gooch.

Dislocated and dislocatable hips in the newborn: the ultrasound scans were provided courtesy of Dr Dennis Remedios and the photographs of the Pavlik harness courtesy of Mr L Freedman.

For all photographs apart from those mentioned specifically above, Dr H B Valman and Dr R M Thomas retain the copyright. We thank Mr R Lamont for providing extensive new material for the chapter on prenatal assessment. We are indebted to the Child Growth Foundation for allowing the use of data to construct the growth chart on page 70 and the BMI chart on page 85.

We thank Arlene Baroda for advice on testing for defects in hearing.

CHAPTER 1

Prenatal Assessment

OVERVIEW

- All pregnant women are offered antenatal screening tests after explanation
- Some screening tests provide an assessment of risk (e.g. for Down syndrome) rather than confirmation or exclusion of a diagnosis
- Ultrasound scanning does not exclude all congenital anomalies
- Preterm labour is often associated with maternal infection

Box 1.2 **First antenatal visit – routine blood screening**

- Full blood count and haemoglobin electrophoresis
- Blood group
- Rhesus antibody titre
- Rubella antibody status
- Hepatitis B antibodies
- HIV antibodies
- Syphilis serology

Recent advances in ultrasound technique, equipment and training, together with rapid advances in molecular biology have increased the range of antenatal diagnoses (Box 1.1). Some methods are available only at specialized centres. This chapter will give a background to successful techniques.

An anomaly may be detected during routine examination of the fetus which is carried out by ultrasound between 18 and 20 weeks of gestation. The risk of the most common chromosomal anomaly, Down syndrome, can be evaluated by several methods.

After the birth of an abnormal baby or the detection of genetic disease in an older child, a paediatrician or geneticist may recommend a specific test at a particular week in the subsequent pregnancy. Some tests are at an early stage in development and the false positive and negative rates have not been assessed. Some genetic tests are not yet sufficiently precise to enable an accurate prognosis to be given to every family with that disease.

At the first antenatal visit it is still important to carry out a full blood count and haemoglobin electrophoresis, blood grouping, rhesus antibody titre, and tests for rubella, hepatitis B,

Box 1.1 **Routine screening**

- Ultrasound scan for gestational age assessment at 11–14 weeks
- Detailed anomaly ultrasound scan at 18–20 weeks
- Combined screening test for Down syndrome
- Routine blood screening

ABC of the First Year, Sixth edition. By B. Valman and R. Thomas. © 2009 Blackwell Publishing, ISBN: 978-1-4051-8037-5.

human immunodeficiency virus (HIV) and syphilis (Box 1.2). The haemoglobin electrophoresis may show that the mother has β-thalassaemia trait or sickle cell trait and the father's red cell investigations may suggest that further studies of the fetus are needed.

Ultrasound studies

The first routine examination of the fetus by ultrasound is usually performed at the gestational age of 11–14 weeks. The gestational age is confirmed and anomalies of the central nervous system or cystic hygromas may be detected. A further scan at 18–20 weeks may detect anomalies of the central nervous system, heart, kidneys, intestinal tract and skeleton (Figure 1.1). Signs that suggest the possibility of a chromosome abnormality include choroid plexus cysts, echogenic cardiac foci, renal pelvic dilatation and echogenic bowel. They occur in approximately 1 in 250 pregnancies and are associated with a 1 in 300 risk of a chromosome abnormality. These isolated 'soft' signs do not merit the fetal risks of amniocentesis, but full discussion is necessary and the mother may still opt for karyotyping to be performed. Mothers with a family history of congenital heart disease should be offered a detailed fetal echocardiogram at 18–24 weeks as the risk of the fetus having a heart problem is 3–5%. The consultant obstetrician or fetal medicine specialist, ideally with the neonatal paediatrician, should discuss the diagnosis and prognosis of an anomaly with both parents. Termination of the pregnancy may need to be considered, or serial ultrasound examination performed during the pregnancy and in the neonatal period.

Ultrasound guidance is used in taking samples of the amniotic fluid (amniocentesis) and in selected centres it has been used to take blood samples from the umbilical cord (cordocentesis) and very occasionally to give blood transfusion by that route.

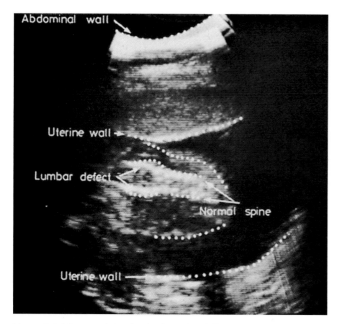

Figure 1.1 Ultrasound showing lumbar spine defect.

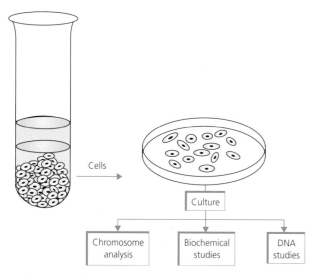

Figure 1.2 Examination of amniotic fluid.

The samples can be used in gene probe techniques, enzyme estimation and chromosome studies. In rhesus incompatibility, a low haematocrit in the cord blood in association with rhesus-negative status of the mother indicates the need for fetal transfusion.

Amniocentesis

Amniotic fluid is removed by passing a needle into the amniotic cavity through the mother's abdominal wall and uterus under ultrasound guidance. Amniocentesis yields amniotic fluid containing cells that have been shed from the skin of the fetus. Examination of the cultured cells reveals the chromosome constitution of the fetus, including sex (Figure 1.2). Specific enzymes can be sought and deoxyribonucleic acid (DNA) probes used (Figure 1.3). Women

Autosomal dominant
- Huntington's chorea
- Myotonic dystrophy
- Adult polycystic kidneys
- Tuberous sclerosis
- Von Recklinghausen's disease

X linked
- Duchenne muscular dystrophy
- Haemophilia A and B
- Fragile X

Autosomal recessive
- α and β-thalassaemia
- Sickle cell disease
- Cystic fibrosis
- Phenylketonuria
- α1-Antitrypsin deficiency
- Congenital adrenal hyperplasia

Figure 1.3 Examples of conditions for which DNA gene probes are available.

who are found to be at higher risk for Down syndrome on a screening test are offered amniocentesis. In high-risk women a fluorescent in situ hybridization (FISH) test may be offered which uses the polymerase chain reaction (PCR) to detect chromosome abnormalities such as the common trisomies 21, 18 and 13 – Down, Edward and Patau syndrome respectively. The results are available within a few working days.

Chorionic villus biopsy

Chorionic villus biopsy is carried out mainly by the transabdominal route under ultrasound guidance after 10 weeks gestation. The main indications are maternal age, previous chromosome anomaly, fetal sexing, enzyme assay and gene probe assessment. Gene probes have been developed for several diseases including cystic fibrosis, Duchenne muscular dystrophy and the haemoglobinopathies. DNA is extracted from the chorionic villus sample and the probe is used to determine whether a specific part of a particular gene is present or absent.

There is a higher miscarriage rate with chorionic villus biopsy compared to amniocentesis. As there is a risk of limb reduction deformities and facial anomalies when it is performed early, it should be carried out after the 10th week of gestation.

Maternal serum screening for Down syndrome

The majority of babies with Down syndrome are born to mothers under the age of 37 years because they form the largest proportion of mothers. Screening for Down syndrome should be offered to all mothers irrespective of maternal age. It provides an assessment of the risk but not a definite diagnosis of Down syndrome. In the UK, pregnant women are offered a screening test which provides a detection rate above 75% and a false positive rate of less than 3%. There are several tests which meet this standard. The combined test in the first trimester (between 11 and 14 weeks gestation) is offered using nuchal translucency measurement, free β-hCG, pregnancy-associated plasma protein A (PAPP-A) and maternal age.

Accurate gestational assessment as well as measurement of nuchal translucency is undertaken by ultrasound scanning and a maternal blood sample taken at the same antenatal visit (see Box 1.3). The most effective and safe method of screening for Down syndrome is by integration of measurements from the first and second trimesters into a single test result (see Box 1.4). The combined test has the advantage of a risk assessment result being available at an earlier stage in gestation than the integrated test and is therefore more likely to be acceptable to parents. Women who do not attend until the second trimester can be offered a quadruple biochemical test with age standardization. It is hoped that in future, with improved techniques of DNA gene replication, it might be possible to karyotype a fetus using fetal cells in the maternal circulation.

Risks

The risk to a particular fetus depends on the gestational age of the fetus, the indication for the procedure and the experience of the operator. The incidence of complications has fallen as skill in the newer techniques has increased. The abortion rates are difficult to assess but Table 1.1 has been compiled from expert advice on the available evidence. The risk of abortion after amniocentesis at 15 weeks is about 1%, which is about twice the spontaneous incidence in normal pregnancies. Fetal or maternal bleeding has been considerably reduced by the use of ultrasound, but a slight

risk of infection remains and the incidence of respiratory distress syndrome and orthopaedic problems, such as talipes, is probably slightly increased in fetuses who have undergone early amniocentesis. Chorionic villus biopsy has a higher risk of abortion of about 5% against a background of spontaneous abortion of 3%. Chorionic villus biopsy carried out at about 10 weeks gestation provides a result early in pregnancy, when termination of the pregnancy is less traumatic and more acceptable for many mothers. Some tests are slightly more accurate when the sample is obtained by amniocentesis. Some investigations can be performed only on a specific sample.

Table 1.1 Risk of abortion.

Procedure	Gestational age performed (weeks)	Spontaneous abortion (%)	Risk of abortion after procedure (%)
Amniocentesis	14–18	0.5	1
Chorionic villus biopsy	>10	2–3	3–5
Cordocentesis	18–20	<1	1–2

Preterm labour

Preterm birth is the major cause of death and disability in babies. The aetiology of preterm labour is multifactorial, but there is increasing evidence to implicate infection as a possible cause in up to 40% of cases. This information may not help once a woman is admitted in preterm labour, since by that time there may be irreversible changes in the cervix. Where the information may be useful is in the prediction and prevention of preterm labour. A few recent studies have reported that abnormal colonization of the vagina in the form of bacterial vaginosis carries an up to fivefold increased risk of the subsequent development of preterm labour and late miscarriage. Whether by reversing this condition it is possible to reduce the incidence of preterm labour and delivery is currently being tested (Figure 1.4).

The fetal fibronectin test in women with suspected preterm labour and intact membranes between 24 and 34 weeks gestation is a useful adjunct to clinical assessment in deciding whether tocolysis or *in utero* transfer to a perinatal centre should be planned. A negative test indicates that the risk of delivery in the next 7 days is less than 1%.

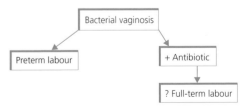

Figure 1.4 Bacterial vaginosis.

Follow-up of fetal renal tract anomalies

Mild dilatation (<10 mm) of the fetal renal pelvis is often found on the routine antenatal ultrasound scan done at 18–20 weeks

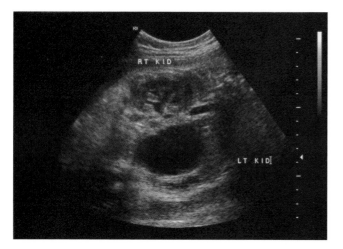

Figure 1.5 Ultrasound scan showing dilatation of left fetal renal pelvis.

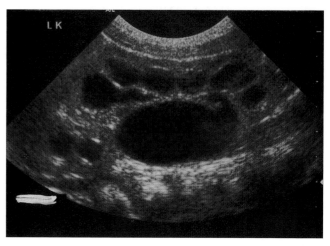

Figure 1.6 Postnatal scan showing dilatation of renal pelvis.

gestation (Figure 1.5). Serial scans at 2–4-weekly intervals will establish whether there is any progressive change before birth. The finding of reduced liquor, a distended thick-walled bladder or progressive dilatation >20 mm may be suggestive of an obstructive uropathy. Preterm delivery or antenatal surgical intervention is rarely indicated, except very occasionally in a male fetus where posterior urethral valves are causing renal compromise at <34 weeks gestation.

For most infants, postnatal investigation with several ultrasound scans over the first few months of life and sometimes a micturating cystourethrogram (MCUG) or renal isotope scan will be necessary. Until the results of these investigations are known, most infants will be given a small daily dose of prophylactic oral antibiotics (usually trimethoprim 1–2 mg/kg). This is to prevent urinary tract infections in those infants who may be at risk because they have vesicoureteric reflux. The radiological investigations are rarely urgent and some are more meaningful when the infant is a little older (for example, isotope scans).

All infants should be followed up postnatally, as it is not easy to predict which infants will have significant ongoing dilatation, but most antenatally diagnosed fetal renal tract dilatation is found to be benign or transient on serial postnatal follow-up (Figure 1.6). A small number of infants will be diagnosed as having pelviureteric junction obstruction, multicystic dysplastic kidney or bladder outlet obstruction, but only the latter requires urgent diagnosis and surgery in the neonatal period.

Further reading

NHS. *Antenatal and newborn screening programmes.* www.nscfa.web.its. manchester.ac.uk/screeninginfo

Royal College of Obstetricians. *Antenatal screening for Down syndrome.* www.rcog.org.uk/resources

Lamont RF (2003) Recent evidence associated with the condition of preterm prelabour rupture of the membranes. *Current Opinion in Obstetrics and Gynaecology* 15: 91–99.

CHAPTER 2

Resuscitation of the Newborn

OVERVIEW

- Most newborn infants do not need resuscitation and respond to stimulation by gentle drying in a warm environment
- Regular training in neonatal resuscitation should be provided for all healthcare workers who are involved in maternity care
- Intubation is rarely needed, but requires a skilled clinician
- Drugs are seldom helpful

Wherever babies are delivered there should be a person with appropriate training and experience in resuscitation immediately available throughout the 24 hours (Box 2.1). The majority of babies do not require resuscitation and those who do can be resuscitated with a closely fitting mask and an inflatable bag with a valve. The equipment is cheap and simple to use, and can be carried in a small case. A very few infants cannot be resuscitated by this method and will require intubation, which to be successful should be done by a doctor, nurse or midwife with continual experience of the procedure.

Babies who have developmental brain abnormalities before labour may develop fetal distress during the stress of labour and may have difficulty in establishing spontaneous respiration. For this reason, the contributions of brain development and perinatal management in the causation of later cerebral palsy are often difficult to resolve.

Assessment

The following high-risk factors indicate that resuscitation may be needed:

- fetal distress
- preterm delivery
- breech delivery
- forceps delivery
- multiple pregnancy
- maternal general anaesthetic
- maternal diabetes
- cord prolapse
- antepartum haemorrhage.

These factors predict about 70% of the babies needing resuscitation. The remainder arise unexpectedly. The APGAR scoring system is used to assess the infant's condition at 1 minute and 5 minutes after birth (Table 2.1). A numerical score is given for each of five features. The heart rate and respiratory effort determine the action to be taken.

Procedure

Suctioning the oropharynx

The rare indications for suction of the oropharynx are meconium aspiration and blood in the mouth. It is best not to use manual mucus extractors, as there is a risk of the operator swallowing or inhaling potentially infectious material. Use a suction catheter

---

Box 2.1 **Basic neonatal life support**

Keep infant warm and stimulate gently by drying.

If not breathing by 60 seconds or if heart rate <100/min

A – airway – position
B – breathing – inflate the lungs
C – circulation – chest compressions
D – drugs – rarely needed

Table 2.1 APGAR scoring system.

	0	1	2
Appearance (colour)	Blue, pale	Body pink, extremities blue	Completely pink
Pulse (heart rate)	Absent	Below 100	Over 100
Grimace (response to stimulation)	No response	Grimace	Cry
Activity (muscle tone)	Limp	Some flexion in extremities	Active movements
Respiration (respiratory effort)	Absent	Slow irregular	Strong cry

ABC of the First Year, Sixth edition. By B. Valman and R. Thomas. © 2009 Blackwell Publishing, ISBN: 978-1-4051-8037-5.

(size FG 8) connected to a resuscitaire or directly to a wall suction unit. The mouth of the infant can be suctioned safely, but care must be taken in the oropharynx. This should be done under direct vision and is usually part of tracheal intubation. Do not blindly push the catheter as far as it will go, since this can cause a vagally mediated bradycardia and apnoea and is invariably associated with a fall in oxygen saturation.

Administering facial oxygen

Set the oxygen flow rate to 5 L/min and hold the funnel-shaped mask just in front of the baby's face. The oxygen may be connected either to the funnel-shaped mask or to the bag and mask apparatus, but in the case of the latter, it is prevented from flowing out of the mask by the valve unless the bag is compressed. However, it will come out of the corrugated tube that is attached to the other end of the bag, so turn it round and hold the end of this tube to the baby's face. The flow of oxygen to the face will provide a stimulus to breathing, as well as an oxygen-rich environment for the first few breaths.

Using the bag and mask

If the infant does not breathe by 60 seconds after birth or if the heart rate is less than 100/min, the closely fitted mask is applied to the face with the head in the neutral position (Figure 2.1). For a right-handed person, the left hand is used to hold the mask to the baby's face while the right hand squeezes the bag. Place the little and ring fingers of your left hand under the infant's chin, taking care not to push too hard. Alternatively the jaw is elevated with two fingers on the angle of the mandible. This prevents the head from moving around and straightens the upper airways, ensuring their patency. With the other fingers and thumb, apply the mask firmly to the infant's face to ensure a tight seal. A proper seal is confirmed when you squeeze the bag, as there is a characteristic rasping noise as the valve opens. If the seal is inadequate, the valve makes no noise and you will not feel any resistance when squeezing the bag. This can be practised with the mask against the palm of your hand. Use only the thumb and two fingers, rather than your whole hand,

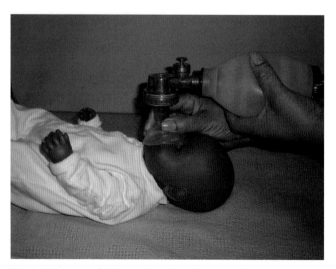

Figure 2.1 Operator holding mask with right hand to show how to place the infant's head in the neutral position.

to squeeze the bag. Do not empty the bag but gently depress it to a few centimetres only. This will safeguard against a pneumothorax. The valve on neonatal resuscitation bags is usually set to allow a maximum pressure of 30 cm of water which is safe for most term infants. Gentler, lower inflation pressures will be adequate for pre-term infants. The first five inflations should be slightly prolonged to around 2 seconds, as lung fluid is still present in the airway. Check that you are producing adequate chest expansion by watching the rise and fall of the chest. The most common problem preventing adequate lung inflation is incorrect positioning of the head and neck, usually overextension which obstructs the airway. Air can be used, but oxygen should be used if it can be introduced into a side arm. Reassess the infant after five inflation breaths. If lung inflation has been successful, the heart rate will be increasing. If the infant is still not beginning to breathe spontaneously, continue lung inflation using the bag and mask with a rate of 30–40/min and an inflation time of approximately 1 second.

Intubation

If there are no spontaneous respiratory movements after several cycles of inflation breaths or if the heart rate remains less than 100 beats/min the infant should be placed supine on a flat surface and endotracheal intubation should be done by an experienced clinician (Box 2.2). A special resuscitation trolley is ideal (Figure 2.2a), but is not essential and any firm flat surface is adequate. The laryngoscope is held in the left hand and passed over the infant's tongue as far as the epiglottis (Figures 2.3 & 2.4a). The tip of the blade is advanced over the epiglottis about another 0.5 cm and is then withdrawn slightly. This presses the epiglottis against the root of the tongue, revealing the glottis (Figure 2.5). In the newborn, the glottis is a slit in the centre of a small pink mound and the slit may expand into a triangular opening during a gasp. Gentle backward pressure on the infant's larynx by an assistant may help to bring the glottis into view. Secretions in the pharynx or trachea should be aspirated with a large catheter (e.g. FG 9). The endotracheal tube held in the right hand is then guided through the larynx about 1–2 cm into the trachea (Figure 2.4a,b & 2.5). A metal introducer inside the endotracheal tube makes introduction easier, but it is essential to ensure that it does not extend beyond the end of the tube.

Intermittent positive pressure should be applied at a rate of 40 times per minute with an inflatable bag with a valve or by occluding the T-piece connected to low-flow oxygen attached to a pressure monitor.

The positive pressure applied should not usually be higher than 30 cmH$_2$O; otherwise there is a danger of rupturing the lung and producing a pneumothorax or pneumomediastinum. These low pressures are enough to induce a gasp reflex, which is then followed by normal respiratory movements of the chest. Occasionally

---

Box 2.2 **Indications for intubation in delivery suite**

- To secure the airway in prolonged resuscitation
- After suctioning meconium from the larynx
- For administration of surfactant if <28 weeks gestation
- Hydrops fetalis

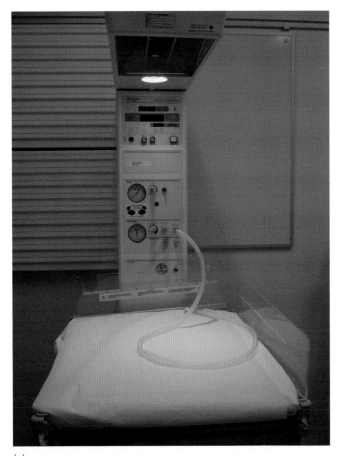

(a)

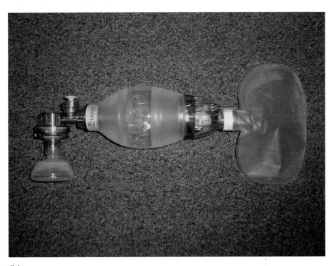

(b)

Figure 2.2 (a) Resuscitation trolley. (b) Bag with face mask.

in an infant with a severe lung problem, such as severe meconium aspiration or diaphragmatic hernia, higher pressures are needed. A return to a normal heart rate is a good sign that resuscitation is satisfactory. If the endotracheal tube has to be left in place for a short period, the tube should be fixed to the cheek by adhesive tape or a special tube holder.

Aspiration of secretions in the endotracheal tube and in the trachea can be carried out with a fine catheter (suction catheter

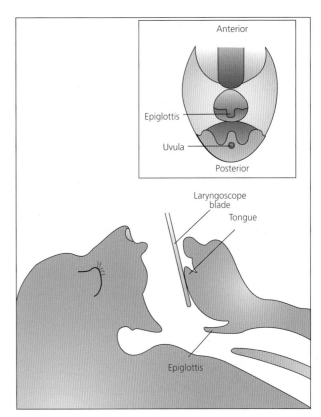

Figure 2.3 Passing the laryngoscope over the tongue.

FG 6). Either a straight or a shouldered tube is satisfactory for emergency resuscitation of the newborn. The shoulder of the endotracheal tube is designed to prevent the tube going too far down through the vocal cords and therefore into the right main bronchus, but this may still occur. If breath sounds are heard equally on both sides of the chest, the tube is probably in the trachea and not beyond the bifurcation.

Intermittent positive pressure should be stopped every 3 minutes for about 15 seconds to determine whether spontaneous respiratory movements will start.

Support the circulation – cardiac compressions

During prolonged apnoea, the blood pressure is maintained initially, but later falls. If the heart rate is less than 100/min, a short period of cardiac massage should be given at the same time as efforts to start respiratory movements. The aim of cardiac compressions in newborn infants is to move oxygenated blood from the pulmonary veins to the coronary arteries. Cardiac massage is carried out by applying firm pressure with two fingers over the lower sternum one finger's breadth below an imaginary line between the two nipples. In small infants, an alternative method is to encircle the thorax with the fingers of both hands interlocked posteriorly and while applying pressure over the lower sternum with both thumbs. The anteroposterior diameter of the chest should be reduced by one-third during each compression. There should be three cardiac compressions followed by one inflation breath (3:1 ratio of compressions to ventilation).

Hypothermia is a special hazard for infants who have been resuscitated and exposed during these procedures. Extremely

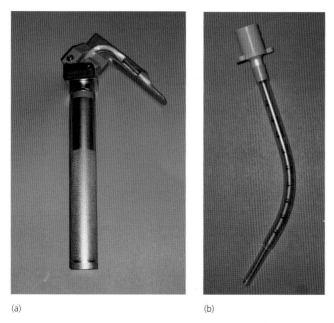

(a)   (b)

Figure 2.4 (a) Small laryngoscope with a straight blade. (b) Neonatal endotracheal tube.

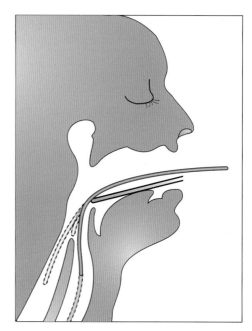

Figure 2.6 Misplacement of the endotracheal tube into the pharynx or oesophagus.

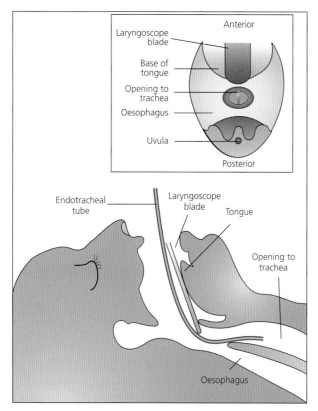

Figure 2.5 Pressing the epiglottis against the root of the tongue.

preterm infants can be placed in a plastic warmer bag without drying and the head covered with a cotton hat immediately after delivery in order to reduce heat loss. Rapid initial drying of the term infant with a warm towel is the most important preventive factor. Resuscitation should also be carried out under a radiant heater of at least 400 W. After resuscitation, infants should be wrapped up and handed to their mothers for at least a few minutes if their response to resuscitation has been satisfactory, even if they have to be placed in a transport incubator and taken to the special care unit. Most full-term infants who have required resuscitation do not need to be admitted to the special care unit.

Failure to improve

The best sign that resuscitation has been successful is an increase in heart rate. If this does not occur within about 15 seconds the following should be considered.

1 The gas cylinders may be empty or the gas tubing has disconnected.
2 The endotracheal tube may have been misplaced into the oesophagus or have slipped out of the trachea during extension of the neck (Figure 2.6).
3 The endotracheal tube may have become blocked with thick secretions e.g. meconium or blood. If there is any doubt and after checking for correct positioning of the head and neck, the tube should be removed and a fresh tube inserted immediately.
4 The endotracheal tube may be in the right main bronchus.

After these possibilities have been excluded, other rare diagnoses to be considered are pneumothorax, pulmonary hypoplasia associated with Potter's syndrome (renal agenesis with a squashed facial appearance and large, low set floppy ears) and diaphragmatic hernia.

Drugs

Ventilation using bag and mask or intubation is usually effective in resuscitation of the newborn and drugs are rarely necessary. Drugs are useless if the lungs have not been inflated. If the infant needs

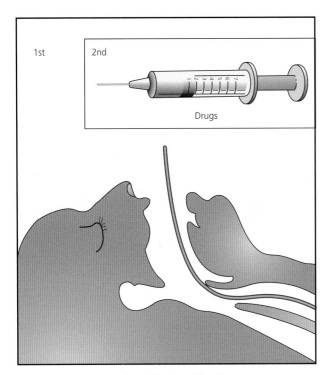

1st 2nd

Drugs

Figure 2.7 Intubation is performed before giving drugs.

Table 2.2 Recommended doses. IC, intracardiac; IT, intratracheal; UVC, umbilical venous catheter.

Drug	Concentration	Route	Dose (mL/kg)	Dose for 3 kg baby (mL)
Adrenaline	1 in 10 000 (0.1 mg/mL)	UVC, IT, rarely IC	0.1 mL/kg	0.3 mL
Sodium bicarbonate	4.2% (8.4% 1 mmol/mL diluted 1:1 with sterile water or 5% or 10% dextrose)	UVC	2–4 mL/kg (diluted 1:1 with water)	6–12 mL
Glucose	10%	UVC	1–2 mL/kg	3–6 mL

both intubation and drugs, intubation should always be performed first (Figure 2.7).

An adequate supply of oxygen quickly reverses acidosis and it is rarely necessary to consider giving intravenous sodium bicarbonate or glucose solution. For recommended doses, see Table 2.2.

If drugs are given, administration via an umbilical venous catheter is usually more appropriate than via a peripheral vein.

Adrenaline can be given if there is asystole or there is persistent severe bradycardia, but there is no evidence that it improves the long-term outcome. The preferred route of administration of adrenaline is via the umbilical vein, but the endotracheal route is effective and may be easier to give. If there is no response, adrenaline can be repeated. Intracardiac adrenaline is rarely desirable. The use of adrenaline, sodium bicarbonate, volume expanders or 0.9% sodium chloride solution is not recommended routinely in the resuscitation of the newborn. Shock in the newborn is usually related to hypoxaemia and responds to administered oxygen, but

a volume expander may be needed where there is volume loss. If there is clear evidence of blood loss 10 mL/kg of 0.9% normal saline is given via the UVC.

A probable acidosis is partially reversed by giving 2–4 mL/kg of 4.2% sodium bicarbonate solution slowly at a rate that does not exceed 2 mL/min. The standard 8.4% sodium bicarbonate solution must be diluted with an equal volume of sterile water or 5% or 10% dextrose. If a glucometer shows hypoglycaemia 1–2 mL/kg of 10% glucose solution can be given.

Calcium is no longer used in newborn resuscitation. Exogenous surfactant is administered prophylactically via the endotracheal route in preterm infants less than 28 weeks gestation in the delivery suite, but it should not be given until the infant has been appropriately resuscitated, is well oxygenated and has a good heart rate. Surfactant is not a drug of resuscitation.

If the mother has recently received pethidine or morphine, a chemical antagonist can be given to the infant if there is no spontaneous breathing after successful resuscitation. The only chemical antagonist available is naloxone, but its period of action is short. The manufacturer's current recommended dose is 10–20 μg/kg given intramuscularly.

Full-term infants in whom there have been significant signs of fetal distress accompanied by significant acidosis, who have a low APGAR score of less than 5 at 5 minutes and who have required resuscitation are at risk of hypoxic ischaemic encephalopathy and cerebral oedema. Cerebral function monitoring over the first 4 hours after birth will help to identify infants at highest risk who may benefit from transfer to a specialist centre for carefully controlled therapeutic total body cooling to improve long-term outcome. The infant may be apnoeic and need continuous positive pressure ventilation, have fits, episodes of bradycardia or lethargy, or be reluctant to suck. Mannitol, frusemide, steroids and phenobarbitone in high doses have been used to prevent or treat possible cerebral oedema, but there is no evidence that they are effective.

These infants will also need long-term follow-up to assess neurological development. MRI brain scan performed at least 4–5 days after birth gives a good indication of long-term prognosis. The survival rate of full-term newborn infants who have taken 20 minutes to breathe spontaneously is about 50%, and about 75% of the survivors are neurologically intact.

When to stop

Poor outcome can be predicted when there is no return of a normal heart rate >120/min and spontaneous respirations are not established by 20–30 minutes. If, in addition, there is no cardiac output, then survival cannot be expected. It is at this stage that attempts at resuscitation should cease.

When not to start

This can be an extremely difficult decision and should not be made by the most junior paediatrician, so begin resuscitation and call for help. If the heart rate has been recorded at any time during the second stage of labour, resuscitation should be attempted even if there is no heartbeat at birth. With fetal monitoring it is uncommon for

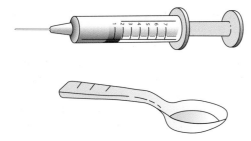

Figure 2.8 Vitamin K may be given intramuscularly or orally.

babies to die during labour and stillbirths are usually expected. Babies who have been dead for longer than 12 hours have an obvious 'macerated' appearance with gross peeling of the skin.

A baby born at less than 22 weeks gestation cannot survive and often a paediatrician will not be called if the obstetrician is sure of the dates. Certain conditions are non-viable, such as anencephaly or gross hydrocephalus, but fortunately these are usually detected prior to birth and a decision is reached with the parents before delivery.

Discussion with parents

An infant who is breathing normally should be given to the mother after a rapid examination. She should be told that the infant seems to be normal and that it is common for infants to need help with breathing at birth. It is important to emphasize that the infant's progress will be no different from that of other infants who have not needed resuscitation. Most infants who have required intubation should go with their mothers to the postnatal wards and receive routine observation. Only if there has been a prolonged period before the establishment of spontaneous respiration should the infant be taken to the special care unit.

Vitamin K

Vitamin K is given to all babies as prophylaxis against haemorrhagic disease of the newborn and is usually administered in the delivery suite. More predictable blood levels are produced by intramuscular compared to oral vitamin K (Figure 2.8). A single intramuscular dose protects against the early form of haemorrhagic disease, which occurs between the second and fourth day, and the late form, which occurs after 3 or 4 weeks. Following controversy on the safety of the intramuscular route, some paediatricians recommend that breastfed babies receive oral vitamin K in the neonatal period and during the subsequent 2 months. Infants receiving a commercial cows' milk preparation exclusively have an adequate intake of vitamin K.

When an infant dies

If resuscitation of an infant has not been successful, the most senior clinician involved, preferably accompanied by a midwife or nurse, should see the parents immediately to impart the news in a sensitive manner (Figure 2.9). The parents should be given as much factual information as is known to the clinicians at the time about the

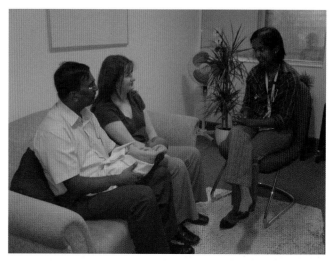

Figure 2.9 Discussion with parents.

likely cause of the death. It should also be made clear that further discussion will need to take place, particularly if the death is sudden or unexpected. The term 'birth asphyxia' should not be used as it may be misleading and there is increasing evidence that neonatal deaths and morbidity are more likely to be due to developmental brain problems or antenatal insults rather than problems occurring during birth. The family doctor should be informed of the death by telephone as soon as possible.

Parents should be encouraged to spend as much time as they want with their infant after death and should be supported by an experienced nurse or midwife. An infant with severe congenital anomalies can be suitably wrapped for the parents to cuddle. Many parents appreciate being able to see the anomalies with a supportive clinician present to discuss any questions they may have at the time. Other family members, including siblings and grandparents, should also be encouraged to see the dead infant over the next few hours or days. It is now clear that the grieving process is helped by family participation in seeing and cuddling their dead infant. Many parents also welcome the opportunity to participate in the care of their dead infant by bathing and dressing the infant in baby clothes of their choice with the assistance of a sympathetic and unhurried nurse. However, healthcare professionals should also be aware that there may be cultural and religious differences that should be respected if parents decline involvement in such procedures after the death of their baby.

Photographs of the dead infant and the family group together with the infant should be encouraged. Photographs should be kept in a safe place if the family do not want to take them away with them immediately, and they may still request them, sometimes even many years later. Hand and footprints and a lock of hair can also be taken as lasting and tangible mementoes for the family.

Discussion with parents will help to decide who will be best able to help the grieving family. There may be a supportive network of family and friends and for some, religious advisers or bereavement counsellors may provide support. If the death occurs in hospital, the family doctor and health visitor should be informed as soon as possible as they will have an important role in supporting the bereaved family in the long term. Siblings should be able to see the dead baby with their parents and should be reassured that they are loved, safe and not in any way to blame for the distress of the parents. Children can accept the death of a baby in a very matter of fact way if they are allowed to be involved and are not excluded from the family at the time of the death. Expert help is rarely necessary for siblings with whom there has been communication and involvement in a manner that is understandable to the child in the bereaved family.

The potential benefits of a postmortem examination should be discussed with the parents by a senior doctor, preferably a consultant. The nature of the autopsy process should be explained in a sympathetic but factual manner and parents should be aware of the possibility of a limited examination of certain body cavities or organs if they do not want to contemplate a full examination. They should be made aware that the face of the baby will not usually be disfigured by the autopsy and that the body can be viewed again later, suitably clothed.

It is important that a healthcare professional with knowledge of the local arrangements for the burial and cremation of infants is available to meet with the parents within a few days of the death in order to assist them to decide how they wish to proceed with funeral arrangements. Although there is a legal requirement to register the death of a baby within 5 working days of the death in the UK, the funeral does not have to take place immediately unless it is a requirement of the religious beliefs of the family. Some families prefer to take some time to decide about arrangements, particularly when the mother of the infant may not be able to be present immediately after a difficult birth.

A follow-up bereavement appointment should be arranged with the parents some weeks later. The results of the postmortem examination should be conveyed to them and they should be given the opportunity to ask questions about the illness and death of their infant. It is usually helpful to parents if the clinicians, including obstetricians or midwives who were present at the birth or involved in the care of the infant, can attend this bereavement discussion. An assessment of whether the family are likely to need expert help and support to progress with their bereavement can also be made at this time. Some parents may also find it helpful to talk to other bereaved families or voluntary organizations providing support, for example SANDS (Stillbirth and Neonatal Death Society).

Further reading

Resuscitation Council UK. (2006) *Newborn Life Support Provider Course Manual: Resuscitation at Birth*, 2nd edn. Resuscitation Council UK, London.

CHAPTER 3

Infants of Low Birthweight

OVERVIEW

- Ten per cent of newborn infants are of low birthweight and most require admission to a neonatal unit for supportive care. Some healthy infants of 34–37 weeks gestation or growth-restricted infants of birthweight >1700 g can be cared for on the postnatal ward with their mother
- Most preterm infants are able to be discharged home around the expected date of birth. They need to be feeding and gaining weight well and be able to maintain a stable temperature, but do not have to be a particular weight or age
- With optimal care, preterm infants born at or above 28 weeks gestation have survival rates and developmental outcomes comparable to full-term infants
- A high proportion of extremely preterm infants <26 weeks gestation have behavioural and learning difficulties by 10 years of age

Low birthweight infants weigh 2500 g or less at birth. Infants may be small at birth owing to a short gestation period (born too early) or because of a restricted intrauterine growth rate (Box 3.1). When the period of gestation is less than 37 completed weeks the infant is called preterm. A baby with restricted growth rate is 'light for dates' or small for gestational age (SGA) and may be either malnourished or pathologically small or hypoplastic; for example, an infant with a chromosome abnormality. Some babies who are preterm are also light for dates (Figure 3.1).

The length of gestation can be calculated from the first day of the mother's last menstrual period, provided the periods are regular. The routine ultrasound examination carried out before

Box 3.1 **Causes of low birthweight (<2500 g)**

- Prematurity – less than 37 completed weeks of gestation
- Intrauterine growth restriction
    malnutrition
    pathological e.g. chromosomal anomaly

ABC of the First Year, Sixth edition. By B. Valman and R. Thomas. © 2009 Blackwell Publishing, ISBN: 978-1-4051-8037-5.

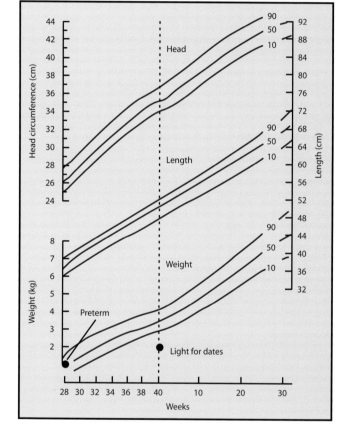

Figure 3.1 Growth chart showing birthweights of preterm and light for dates infants.

18 weeks is considered to be the most accurate method of assessing gestational age. Detecting restriction in growth of the fetus is difficult, but palpation of the fetus can be supplemented by serial ultrasound measurements of the fetal skull, abdominal girth, femur length and crown–rump length.

Gestational age can be assessed by a detailed neurological examination of the infant, as the development of the central nervous system is related to gestational age. Scoring systems using both the neurological development and specific external features (e.g. Dubowitz assessment) can be used to estimate the gestational age but require considerable experience for accuracy.

Most neonatal units consider that infants with a birthweight below the 10th centile for the gestational age are light for dates, although a more accurate definition is below the third centile with an adjustment for maternal size.

Ultrasound studies have shown that when intrauterine malnutrition starts early in pregnancy the head circumference and weight are in proportion with each other, but when malnutrition starts late in pregnancy the head is disproportionately larger than the weight, owing to relatively normal growth of the brain.

The preterm infant is especially prone to developing hypothermia, respiratory distress syndrome, infection and intracranial haemorrhage (Box 3.2). The light for dates infant is particularly prone to hypothermia, hypoglycaemia and hypocalcaemia (Box 3.3).

Temperature

Small infants become hypothermic quickly. Heat loss may be considerable because they have a large surface area in relation to body weight and they are also deficient in subcutaneous fat, which provides insulation. They also lack 'brown fat', which is usually present in a full-term baby and can be metabolized rapidly to produce heat (Figure 3.2).

Hypothermia is associated with a raised metabolic rate and increased energy consumption. To prevent hypothermia, small infants should be kept in a high constant environmental temperature. Excessive heat loss by radiation can be minimized by an additional tunnel of Perspex, a heat shield, placed immediately over an infant in an incubator. Extremely preterm infants can be placed in a plastic warmer bag (Figure 3.4) and the head covered with a cotton hat immediately after delivery in order to reduce heat loss. The dangers of hypothermia can be reduced by carrying out resuscitation under a heat lamp or radiation heat canopy, bearing in mind the danger of burns if the lamp is too close. When a newborn or low birthweight infant is transferred from one hospital to another for specialized care, a portable transport incubator should be used.

The portable incubator must be kept warm continuously and ready for immediate use (Figure 3.3).

Infection

A separate plastic apron or waterproof gown should be used for nursing each infant, mainly to prevent soiling the nurse's clothes.

Scrupulous washing of the hands should be carried out before and after touching each infant. Washing with soap and water is adequate, although many units use a disinfectant soap solution. Scrubbing with a brush is unnecessary. Antiseptic alcohol gel can

---

Box 3.2 **Associations of prematurity**

- Surfactant deficiency
- Respiratory distress syndrome
- Poor temperature regulation
- Risk of infection
- Feeding difficulties
- Periventricular haemorrhage

Box 3.3 **Associations of intrauterine growth restriction**

- Hypothermia
- Hypoglycaemia
- Hypocalcaemia

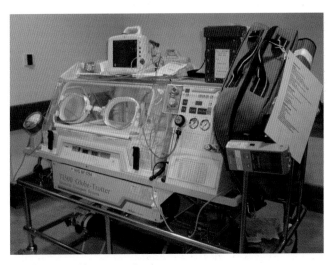

Figure 3.3 Portable transport incubator.

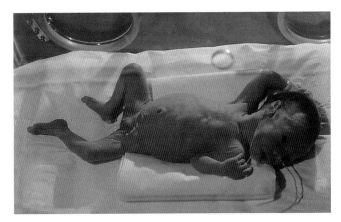

Figure 3.2 Light for dates: 1800 g at 40 weeks.

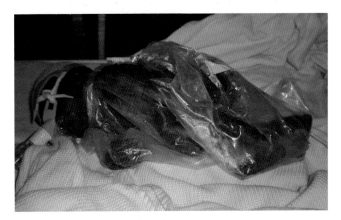

Figure 3.4 Preterm infant in plastic bag.

also be used before and after handling each infant. Although the principle of handwashing is simple, it may be difficult to ensure that it is carried out by all healthcare professionals. Proper use of elbow taps is often difficult because of their poor design. Using disposable plastic gloves when changing infants' napkins may reduce cross-infection.

Thorough handwashing (Figure 3.5) or appropriate use of alcohol gel is generally regarded as adequate for prevention of nosocomial infection, and barrier nursing in a separate cubicle is rarely necessary.

Feeding

Preterm infants have poor sucking and cough reflexes and methods of feeding must prevent aspiration into the lungs. Infants who are not able to suck are given frequent tube feeds of small volumes to avoid sudden falls in arterial oxygen concentration and apnoeic attacks, which are associated with abdominal distension. Orogastric rather than nasogastric tubes are preferred in order not to obstruct the upper airway, but may be more difficult to secure. Intravenous feeding with glucose amino acid solutions and lipids is used for infants who do not tolerate tube feeding, but a scrupulous aseptic technique in managing the solutions is necessary to avoid septicaemia.

Early feeding, as soon as possible and at least within 2 hours of birth, prevents hypoglycaemia and reduces the maximum plasma bilirubin concentrations. Asymptomatic hypoglycaemia can be detected by performing regular blood glucose measurements using a glucometer on all babies of low birthweight in the first 24 hours. If the infant is feeding well and the blood glucose level is consistently above 2.6 mmol/L, the tests are stopped after 24 hours. Once enteral feeds are established, vitamin supplements are added so that infants receive an additional dose of 400 units of vitamin D and 50 mg of vitamin C daily. Vitamin preparations usually contain small amounts of vitamin B complex and vitamin A. Vitamin supplements should be given until the age of 2 years and additional iron supplements until the age of 6 months.

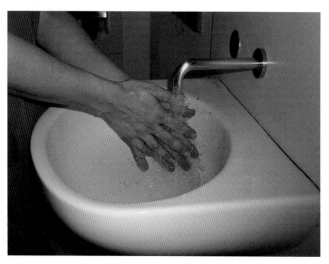

Figure 3.5 Handwashing prevents cross-infection.

The low birthweight infant at home

As more extremely low birthweight infants are surviving, community health professionals need to be aware of a few specific needs and problems of these infants in the first year of life.

Sleep position

Preterm infants are often nursed in the prone position in the neonatal unit as this has been shown to improve oxygenation and reduce apnoeic episodes. By around 36–37 weeks gestation, the sleep position of the infant should have been changed to sleeping on the back in preparation for discharge home, and the benefits of back sleeping in healthy mature infants should be explained to the parents. Very occasionally, side sleeping may be recommended if there is micrognathia or severe gastro-oesophageal reflux. Respiratory monitors and oxygen saturation probes should also be removed in the weeks preceding discharge home, so that parental confidence can be achieved in assessing their baby and so that they do not become reliant on unnecessary monitors.

Home oxygen

Infants who still require a small amount of oxygen but who are feeding and are otherwise well, can often be cared for at home by their parents. An oxygen concentrator for use at home can be prescribed as the continuous provision of oxygen cylinders is impractical in the long term. A small portable cylinder which can be carried on a pram or pushchair will be useful to enable the infant to accompany the family on brief trips outside the home environment.

A community neonatal or paediatric nurse will support the family at home and will monitor the oxygen saturation (Figure 3.6) of the infant intermittently until no additional oxygen is required, sometimes weeks or even months after discharge from hospital. Family carers will have been taught basic life support by the community nurse.

Respiratory problems

Preterm infants, particularly those who have required artificial ventilation, have an increased risk of respiratory illnesses in the first year of life. Wheezing is common in association with viral infections, but only those infants with a strong family history of atopy have an increased incidence of asthma. Smoking should be strongly discouraged in homes where there is a preterm infant.

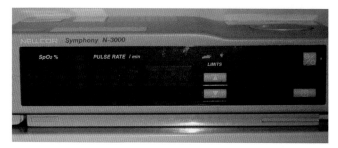

Figure 3.6 Oximeter for measuring blood oxygen saturation.

> **Box 3.4 Supplements for preterm infants**
> - Vitamins A, B, C and D until 2 years of age
> - Phosphate in the first year for extremely preterm infants
> - Iron from 4 weeks to 6 months

Immunizations

Routine immunization with DTaP/IPV/Hib and PCV (diphtheria, tetanus, acellular pertussis/inactivated polio vaccine/*Haemophilus influenzae* and pneumococcal vaccines) can be commenced 8 weeks after birth, irrespective of the gestational age of the infant. Even infants of very early gestation have been shown to mount an appropriate immune response to childhood vaccines. In practice, many preterm infants will still be in the neonatal unit at 2 months of age and some will have had their immunizations commenced before discharge from hospital. Meningococcal C vaccination is commenced at 12 weeks of age. Neonatal BCG immunization is advisable in populations with a high prevalence of tuberculosis.

Vitamins and iron supplementation

Preterm infants require vitamin A, B, C and D supplementation until 2 years of age (Box 3.4). Some extremely immature infants may also require additional phosphate for adequate bone mineralization during the period of rapid growth in the first year of life.

Additional oral iron is usually given from 4 weeks to 6 months of age.

Routine screening tests for preterm and low birthweight infants

Preterm infants <31 weeks gestation or <1500 g birthweight are at risk of retinopathy of prematurity (ROP) and will have routine fundoscopy performed by an ophthalmologist from 6 weeks of age until term. Laser therapy may occasionally be required if there are significant signs of ROP and is usually successful in preventing visual impairment.

All infants have routine audiological screening within the newborn period, and in preterm infants this should be performed at around term.

Blood spot screening for phenylketonuria, hypothyroidism and cystic fibrosis is undertaken at 5–7 days of age in all newborns, and in preterm infants it is repeated again at 36 weeks gestation.

Growth and development

The growth and development of preterm infants born at <30 weeks gestation should be assessed according to their corrected age

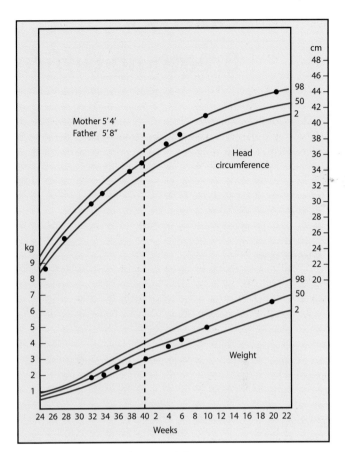

Figure 3.7 Growth chart of a preterm infant.

(chronological age – period of prematurity). Most will have caught up with their peers born at full term by around 18 months to 2 years of age (Figure 3.7). Some extremely low birthweight infants, particularly those born at <26 weeks gestation, remain below the third centile in all growth parameters despite being otherwise healthy. Around 90% of infants <28 weeks gestation who survive to go home achieve normal developmental milestones for their corrected age, but many experience minor motor and educational difficulties by school age. Myopia is also common in children who were preterm.

Further reading

Rennie JM. (2005) *Robertson's Textbook of Neonatology*, 4th edn. Churchill Livingstone, Edinburgh.

CHAPTER 4

Breathing Difficulties in the Newborn

OVERVIEW

- Mild breathing difficulty, particularly tachypnoea 60–80 breaths/min, is common in the first few hours after birth, particularly in infants who are born by caesarean section before the onset of labour. Transient tachypnoea of the newborn (TTN) is usually due to delay in reabsorption of lung liquid which is accelerated by maternal catecholamine secretion in labour

- A small number of infants will have tachypnoea as the presenting symptom of potentially life-threatening early-onset group B streptococcal disease and this cannot be diagnosed on clinical examination, chest radiograph or rapid laboratory tests

- All newborn infants with persistent respiratory symptoms require intravenous antibiotics until blood cultures are proven to be negative

- Non-pulmonary causes of respiratory distress include hypothermia, hyperthermia, hypoglycaemia and metabolic acidosis

Breathing difficulties in the newborn are called respiratory distress (Box 4.1). One or more of the following features are present:

- respiratory rate over 60/min
- an expiratory grunt
- subcostal or intercostal recession or sternal retraction
- cyanosis.

Box 4.1 **Common causes of respiratory distress in the newborn**

- Transient tachypnoea of the newborn
- Surfactant deficiency – respiratory distress syndrome
- Air leaks e.g. pneumothorax
- Meconium aspiration syndrome
- Group B streptococcal pneumonia
- Diaphragmatic hernia
- Congenital heart disease

ABC of the First Year, Sixth edition. By B. Valman and R. Thomas. © 2009 Blackwell Publishing, ISBN: 978-1-4051-8037-5.

Respiratory distress syndrome

The respiratory distress syndrome (hyaline membrane disease) is the commonest cause of respiratory problems in preterm infants. Cerebral ischaemia and haemorrhage, or lung damage, may occur in the acute phase and cause death or long-term morbidity. Hypoxaemia before, during or after birth is a predisposing factor.

The cause is a deficiency of pulmonary surfactant, a substance normally produced by type 2 pneumatocytes and present on the alveolar walls. Surfactant lowers the surface tension in the alveoli so that during the first few breaths the same pressure is required to inflate them all. This produces uniform inflation of all alveoli. Surfactant also prevents the alveolar walls from collapsing during expiration. Without surfactant, the surface tension is great in the smaller alveoli, causing them to collapse, while large alveoli continue to expand easily. Thus there is uneven expansion, with increasingly widespread alveolar collapse (Figure 4.1). Surfactant production in the fetal lung increases with gestational age and reaches adequate levels for normal lung function by about the 36th week. At 27–31 weeks, 35–50% of all infants are affected by the respiratory distress syndrome. The use of antenatal steroids given to the mother has reduced this prevalence in infants of less than 36 weeks gestation.

Microscopy of postmortem specimens of the lungs of preterm infants often shows the presence of amorphous material lining the

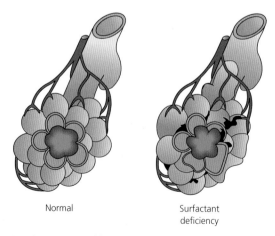

Normal   Surfactant deficiency

Figure 4.1 Cross-section of lungs showing uneven expansion with alveolar collapse in the surfactant-deficient lung.

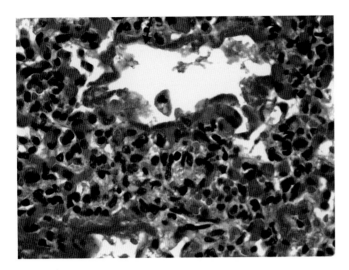

Figure 4.2 Arrow indicates hyaline membrane.

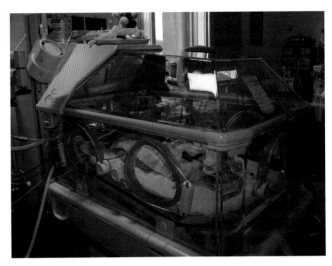

Figure 4.3 Intensive care in a closed incubator.

terminal bronchioles and alveoli, which is called hyaline membrane (Figure 4.2). There are also multiple areas of alveolar collapse.

When animal surfactant extract or artificial surfactant is placed in the trachea via an endotracheal tube soon after birth or during the first few days of life, the severity and mortality of the respiratory distress syndrome are reduced. Supplementary surfactant has been shown to be effective in babies of more than 26 weeks gestation. Supplementary surfactant is given within the first hour after birth to all babies less than 28 weeks gestation (prophylactic treatment) and to more mature infants who have developed features of surfactant deficiency suggesting that the course of the disease will be of moderate or greater severity (rescue treatment).

Clinical features and general management

An expiratory grunt, a respiratory rate over 60/min and recession of the chest wall begin within 4 hours of birth. Central cyanosis may appear if the oxygenation saturation of the blood is not closely monitored. Usually auscultation of the lungs reveals only reduced breath sounds, but crepitations may be present. The current approach to intensive care is to monitor the blood arterial oxygen, carbon dioxide and pH levels from birth, and to start treatment early. This may prevent the appearance of the features described above, especially where artificial ventilation is used electively from birth in infants of less than 28 weeks gestation.

In most infants the chest radiograph shows normal lung fields in the early stages of the disease, but later a fine reticular pattern or generalized loss of translucency (the ground glass appearance) may be present. The contrast between the air in the bronchi and the opaque lung fields produces an air bronchogram. The chest radiograph will be modified or may appear normal in infants who are ventilated and have received exogenous surfactant. The greatest value of the chest radiograph is in excluding other conditions such as air leaks (see below).

The aim of management is to support infants until natural surfactant is produced, a process which usually starts within 48–72 hours of birth, irrespective of the gestation. Infants should be handled as little as possible, as their condition may deteriorate abruptly (Figure 4.3). Elective monitoring of blood oxygen

---

Box 4.2 **Management of respiratory distress syndrome**

- Temperature control
- Prophylactic surfactant if <28 weeks gestation
- Maintain arterial oxygen, carbon dioxide and pH
- Rescue surfactant if ventilated
- Maintain blood pressure
- Fluid and electrolyte balance

---

saturation, heart rate, temperature and respiratory rate has reduced the need to handle the infant. Infants should be given oxygen, their arterial blood oxygen and carbon dioxide concentrations should be monitored, and body temperature, fluid and electrolyte balance maintained (Box 4.2).

Oxygen treatment and measurement

During oxygen treatment the arterial oxygen tension should not fall below 6–7 kPa (50 mmHg) or rise above 12 kPa (90 mmHg). Below 6.7 kPa, the risk of cerebral palsy and mental impairment increases, and above 12 kPa there is the possibility of retinopathy of prematurity (ROP) and subsequent blindness. Some infants may need high concentrations of inhaled oxygen to prevent hypoxaemia. This can be given safely with continuous monitoring of oxygen saturation and frequent estimations of the arterial blood oxygen concentrations.

The ideal arterial carbon dioxide level is 5–7 kPa (37.5–52 mmHg). Lower carbon dioxide levels may cause cerebral artery constriction and reduce cerebral blood flow. Higher carbon dioxide levels may lead to cerebral artery dilatation, followed by systemic hypotension or intraventricular haemorrhage.

There are several methods of measuring oxygen concentrations in the blood. Firstly, samples can be taken from an indwelling umbilical or peripheral artery catheter at regular intervals. Secondly, an infrared transducer placed on the skin over a peripheral artery can give continuous recordings of arterial oxygen saturation. This is a very sensitive method of monitoring oxygenation of the blood which demonstrates changes very rapidly, but care must be taken to ensure that saturation levels do not exceed 95%. High levels of oxygen saturation may be associated with potentially dangerous levels of oxygen in the blood. Thirdly, a heated transcutaneous oxygen and carbon dioxide electrode which increases the blood flow to the skin can be used, and the gas tensions measured. The electrode must be moved every 4 hours to avoid burns. The method is non-invasive and the electrode is calibrated with a gas mixture.

The levels shown by the transcutaneous electrode or saturation monitor must be compared with levels estimated in arterial blood at regular intervals (Figure 4.4). The blood samples are also used to measure pH, bicarbonate and base deficit. Capillary heel prick samples for blood gas analysis are used in infants of greater than 31 weeks gestation in whom the risk of ROP is low, but correlation with arterial blood samples is variable.

Artificial ventilation

Results of artificial ventilation have improved considerably and deaths are now usually due to complications rather than respiratory failure (Figure 4.5). Respiratory tract infection and displacement

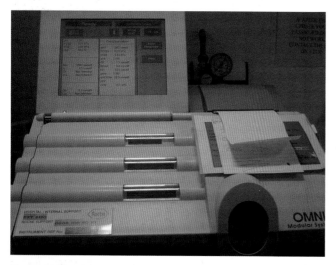

Figure 4.4 Blood oxygen analyser.

of the endotracheal tube are constant hazards and this form of treatment can only be undertaken where there are adequate nursing and medical staff and enough patients for skills to be maintained and an effective service provided. Some neonatal units prefer to use early continuous positive airway pressure (CPAP) via nasal cannulae in order to try to reduce the need for artificial ventilation.

Positive pressure ventilation is needed if one of the following is present:

- failure to establish effective spontaneous respiration at birth
- recurrent apnoeic attacks
- arterial oxygen tension (PaO_2) less than 7 kPa in 60% oxygen
- arterial carbon dioxide tension ($PaCO_2$) more than 7 kPa
- rapid deterioration in blood gas values associated with clinical deterioration.

Other aspects of treatment

Incubators are used to improve observation and to provide warmth and humidified air. Adequate fluids and electrolytes must be given and urine output monitored. The methods of fluid administration will vary with the severity of the respiratory problem. Small volumes of milk can be given intermittently at frequent intervals. The mother's own expressed breast milk is best for the infant and usually tolerated better than formula milk. Some infants need intravenous fluids which may include total parenteral nutrition (TPN) which contains glucose, amino acids, lipids and vitamins.

The group B streptococcus may produce a clinical picture similar to that of respiratory distress syndrome and infants with the respiratory distress syndrome are given antibiotics to cover this possibility. Intravenous antibiotics must be given until blood culture results are known, as the syndrome cannot be differentiated from group B streptococcal pneumonia in the early stages.

Complications

A pneumothorax should be suspected in any infant whose condition deteriorates rapidly for no obvious reason. The diagnosis may be confirmed quickly by transilluminating each side of the chest with a powerful fibreoptic light source. A chest radiograph can be used to confirm the condition (Figure 4.6), but if symptoms are

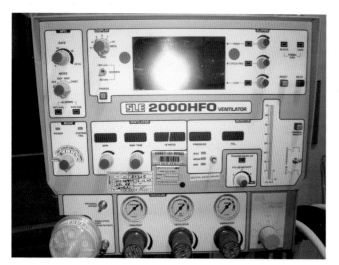

Figure 4.5 Ventilator.

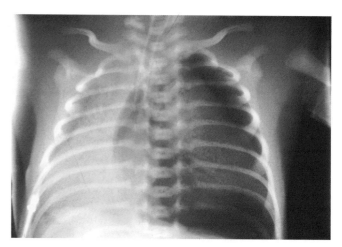

Figure 4.6 Pneumothorax.

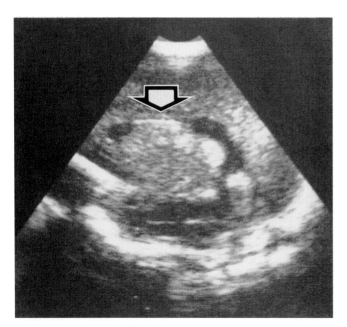

Figure 4.7 Arrow shows intraventricular haemorrhage.

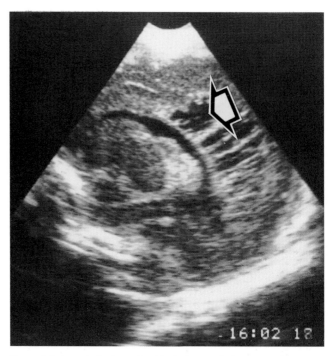

Figure 4.8 Arrow indicates periventricular leucomalacia.

life-threatening, the pneumothorax can be drained before the radiograph has been obtained. A disposable intercostal cannula is inserted into the pleural space and connected to an underwater seal. Pneumothorax may also follow intermittent positive pressure ventilation during resuscitation of the newborn or it may occur as a result of the initial vigorous spontaneous respiratory efforts of a normal infant. Air in the mediastinum (pneumomediastinum) is a common air leak which often precedes the development of a pneumothorax, but pneumomediastinum rarely causes any symptoms and does not require drainage.

Cerebral lesions

Periventricular haemorrhage is the most common form of haemorrhage in the newborn infant (Figure 4.7). Advances in neonatal care have led to increased survival of preterm infants who are susceptible to periventricular haemorrhage. When ultrasound scans have been performed routinely within the first few days of life about 10% of infants with a birthweight less than 1500 g have evidence of periventricular haemorrhage. The majority of these haemorrhages are small and localized and are associated with a good prognosis, but early mortality is high and long-term disability is common in infants with extensive haemorrhages. These haemorrhages originate in the subependymal germinal matrix and may spread to involve the ventricular system or may extend into the cerebral parenchyma adjacent to the lateral ventricle. Most of the infants with periventricular haemorrhage have no specific symptoms but some have recurrent apnoeic attacks, impaired spontaneous limb movements and hypotonia or sudden severe clinical deterioration.

Periventricular leucomalacia is considered to be related to hypoxaemia and ischaemia of the brain. Cysts may develop in areas of haemorrhagic infarction in the periventricular region

and can be shown in ultrasound scans of the brain taken after the third week of life (Figure 4.8). These lesions are associated with later major disabilities such as cerebral palsy, blindness or deafness.

About 15% of infants who survive the neonatal period have some degree of developmental problem and about 7% have a severe problem. Surviving infants of less than 26 weeks gestation have a higher risk of neurodevelopmental and behavioural problems.

Chronic lung disease (bronchopulmonary dysplasia)

This is a chronic respiratory disease occurring in preterm babies who are very preterm or have needed artificial ventilation. The causes are multifactorial and include inflammation, barotrauma from artificial ventilation, recurrent aspiration of milk or post-natal infection. The infant requires increased inflation pressures or ambient oxygen concentrations as coarse streaking and areas of hyperinflation appear on the chest radiograph after the first 2 or 3 weeks of life (Figure 4.9). After weaning from the ventilator, supplementary oxygen is often required for several months and those with severe disease have a high mortality in the first year of life. Survivors have a high prevalence of recurrent episodes of wheezing, but usually have no further clinical respiratory symptoms after about 18 months of age. The duration of oxygen dependency may be reduced by dexamethasone but this is associated with a high risk of cerebral palsy and is used only in infants with life-threatening chronic lung disease and after discussion with the parents about the associated risks. Some infants with long-term oxygen dependency who are otherwise stable are cared for at home by their parents. Evaluation of intermittent overnight saturation monitoring by an experienced community neonatal or paediatric

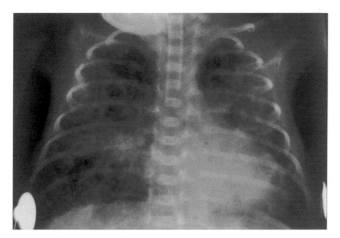

Figure 4.9 Bronchopulmonary dysplasia.

nurse will help in making the decision as to when supplementary oxygen can be discontinued.

Other causes of respiratory problems

The main causes are pulmonary, cardiac and central nervous system disorders.

Transient tachypnoea of the newborn occurs in infants after a short labour or elective caesarean section, before or at term. It can occur in preterm infants but there may be difficulty in distinguishing it from mild respiratory distress syndrome. Transient tachypnoea usually resolves within 48 hours. The chest radiograph often shows a streaky appearance of the lung fields, but may be normal. This syndrome is most likely due to delayed reabsorption of the normal lung fluid at birth.

Diaphragmatic hernia may present with difficulty in resuscitating the baby or with a raised respiratory rate and an apex beat on the right side. The hernia is most commonly left sided and the heart is often displaced to the right. Most diaphragmatic hernias are detected by antenatal ultrasound scans. The diagnosis is confirmed by a chest radiograph that shows loops of small gut or solid organs in the thorax (Figure 4.10). It may take up to 12 hours from birth for air to reach the colon and produce the characteristic radiographic appearances.

The first symptoms of *congenital heart disease* are often noticed by the nurse or mother when the infant has dyspnoea during feeding or is reluctant to feed. There may be no murmurs with some lesions. The respiratory rate is raised and there may be recession of the chest wall. Excessive weight gain and enlargement of the liver are early confirmatory signs. The edge of the liver is normally about 2 cm below the costal margin in the right midclavicular line in the full-term newborn. Cardiomegaly (enlargement of the heart) may be seen on a chest radiograph (Figure 4.11).

Pneumonia may occur if there has been rupture of the membranes for longer than 24 hours: the infant may inhale infected liquor before birth and so develop pneumonia. If the mother has had ruptured membranes for over 18 hours before delivery,

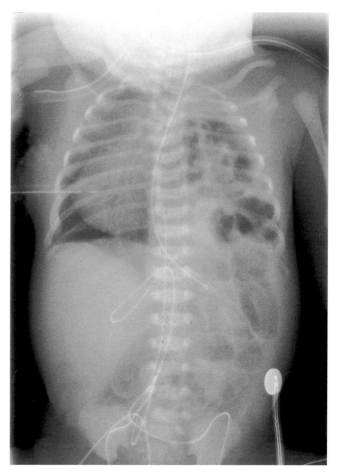

Figure 4.10 Diaphragmatic hernia.

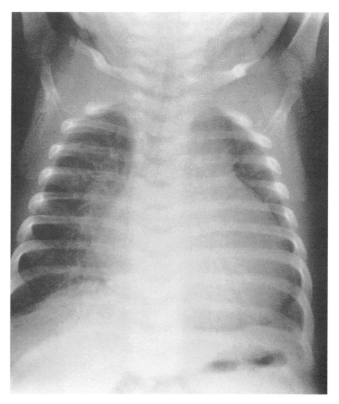

Figure 4.11 Large heart.

antibiotics should be considered for the mother to prevent or treat pneumonia in the fetus.

Group B streptococcal infection may present with a raised respiratory rate and a chest radiograph may show extensive areas of consolidation in both lungs or may appear normal.

Meconium aspiration usually occurs in an infant who has become hypoxic before delivery. The infant may start gasping before the mouth and pharynx have been cleared. Aspiration of meconium may cause bronchial obstruction, secondary collapse and subsequent infection of the distal segments of the lungs. Oxygen and antibiotics are often needed and mechanical ventilation may be required.

Preterm infants have a poor cough reflex and material such as regurgitated milk in the pharynx is easily aspirated into the lungs and may cause pneumonia. Signs may be minimal and are often limited to a small increase in respiratory rate, but a chest radiograph may show extensive changes.

Severe anaemia may cause a raised respiratory rate with a metabolic acidosis.

Choanal atresia or stenosis. A congenital posterior nasal obstruction makes it difficult for newborn infants to breathe, as they depend on a clear nasal airway. An oropharyngeal airway produces immediate improvement and an ENT surgeon should be consulted. The diagnosis can be confirmed quickly by noting the absence of movement of a wisp of cotton wool placed just below the nares.

Apnoea

Apnoeic attacks are defined as episodes of cessation of respiratory movements for more than 10 seconds (Figure 4.12). Apnoea may be due to immaturity, cerebral hypoxia during the perinatal period, hypoxaemia due to the respiratory distress syndrome, hypoglycaemia, septicaemia or meningitis (Box 4.3). An ultrasound scan of the brain may help in determining the presence and site of any intracranial haemorrhage.

Morphine or pethidine given to the mother before delivery may cause apnoea in the newborn.

Recurrent apnoeic episodes are common in preterm infants of less than 32 weeks gestation. The babies are otherwise well and the episodes start when the infants are a few days old. The apnoea may be accompanied by bradycardia and a fall in oxygen saturation levels. Recent research suggests that some episodes are of central and others of laryngeal origin. The diagnosis of apnoea of prematurity can be made only after excluding other causes; which are:
- pulmonary disease
- airway obstruction, for example due to aspiration of feeds
- hypoglycaemia
- hypocalcaemia
- intracranial haemorrhage

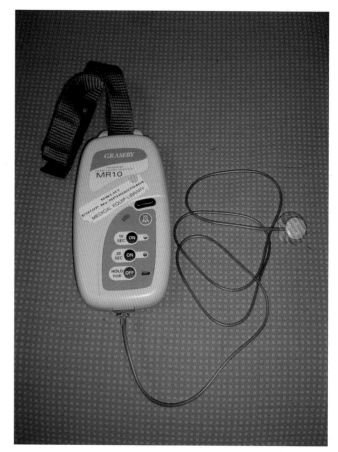

Figure 4.12 Apnoea sensor with alarm.

Box 4.3 **Causes of apnoea**

- Immaturity
- Hypoxia
- Intracranial haemorrhage
- Hypoglycaemia
- Meningitis
- Drugs

- convulsions, which may be misdiagnosed as apnoea
- cardiac disease.

Apnoeic episodes may occur daily up to around 34 weeks gestation. These may be difficult to manage and may be followed by cerebral palsy at a later date if the episodes are prolonged. The various forms of treatment include stimulation of a limb during attacks or prophylaxis with oral caffeine or continuous positive airways pressure.

Further reading

Rennie JM. (2005) *Robertson's Textbook of Neonatology,* 4th edn. Churchill Livingstone, Edinburgh.

CHAPTER 5

Birth Trauma

OVERVIEW

- Mild bruising, swelling and oedema from pressure of the presenting part is extremely common and will resolve spontaneously, but parents need to be reassured about this
- Intracranial haemorrhage is rarely caused by a traumatic delivery and further investigation of the baby may be required

Box 5.1 **Common forms of birth trauma**

- Caput succedaneum
- Cephalhaematoma
- Chignon from vacuum extraction
- Brachial plexus injury (Erb's palsy)
- Facial palsy
- Subconjunctival haemorrhage

Cephalhaematoma

Cephalhaematoma is a subperiosteal haemorrhage that is limited by surrounding sutures (Figure 5.1). In most cases there is probably a hairline fracture of the underlying cranial bone, which may be difficult to demonstrate but is unimportant since it affects only the outer table of the skull. There is usually no brain damage. A surprisingly large amount of blood may be present and blood transfusion is occasionally required. The lesion may not be noticed until the third day. A large cephalhaematoma may be associated with early jaundice or hyperbilirubinaemia.

During resolution a calcified rim may appear, which wrongly suggests a depressed fracture, or there may be a hard swelling that takes several months to disappear.

Cephalhaematoma must be distinguished from caput succedaneum, which is a soft tissue swelling due to oedema of the part of

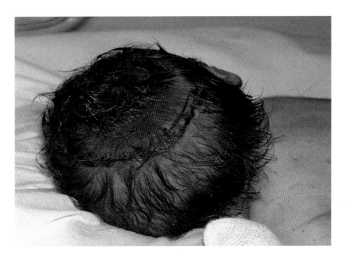

Figure 5.2 Chignon.

the head presenting at the cervix and which is not limited by the sutures (Box 5.1).

Vacuum extraction injuries

Vacuum (ventouse) extraction is often associated with a 'chignon', which is subcutaneous oedema where the cap has been applied (Figure 5.2). In some cases a large haematoma may form and occasionally the skin becomes necrotic. Nevertheless, the skin grows rapidly from the borders to cover the area within a few weeks. Subaponeurotic haemorrhage occasionally occurs and can be life-threatening as it is not limited by the skull sutures, and ongoing significant blood loss continues for up to 24 hours after birth.

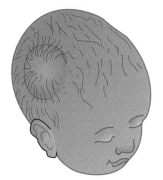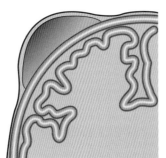

Figure 5.1 Cephalhaematoma.

ABC of the First Year, Sixth edition. By B. Valman and R. Thomas. © 2009 Blackwell Publishing, ISBN: 978-1-4051-8037-5.

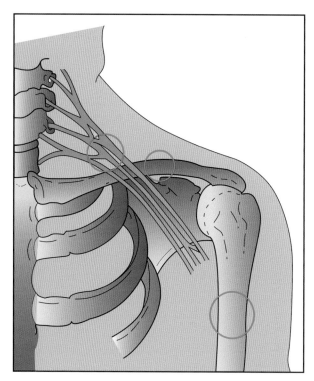

Figure 5.3 Three sites of injury causing reduced arm movements.

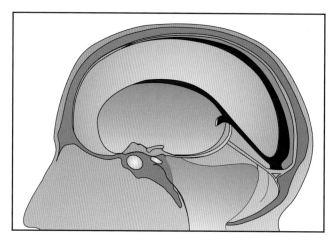

Figure 5.4 Extracerebral haemorrhage may be due to laceration of a venous sinus.

Reduced arm movements

Fractures of the clavicle or humerus and stretching of the brachial plexus present as lack of spontaneous movement and an absent Moro reflex in the arm on that side (Figure 5.3). The clavicle and humerus should be radiographed. Fracture of the clavicle needs no treatment, but if the humerus is fractured the arm should be splinted to the infant's body with a crepe bandage. Injuries to the brachial plexus (Erb's palsy) will be recognized as lack of spontaneous movement of the shoulder and arm with the hand held in dorsiflexion at the wrist (waiter's tip position). Movements of the fingers are associated with good long-term prognosis with spontaneous resolution. Early referral to a physiotherapist and orthopaedic surgeon is advised as injuries to the brachial plexus sometimes have a poor prognosis. Diaphragmatic paralysis may accompany stretching of the brachial plexus and cause a raised respiratory rate. Another condition that may be mistaken for injury of the brachial plexus is temporary paralysis of the dorsiflexors of the wrist caused by pressure on the radial nerve in the radial groove of the humerus. A fracture of the humerus may injure the radial nerve at this site.

Intracranial injuries

When the fetal head is large in relation to the pelvic outlet, or delivery is precipitate or by the breech, there is a risk of extracerebral haemorrhage due to laceration of the tentorium cerebelli or falx cerebri affecting a venous sinus (Figure 5.4).

Infants may be unduly lethargic or especially irritable shortly after birth and there are usually no other helpful confirmatory signs then. Later there may be pallor, a high-pitched cry, poor muscle tone or increased tone, convulsions, reluctance to suck, vomiting, or apnoeic attacks and fast or periodic breathing. Rarely the tension of the anterior fontanelle is raised, the heart rate is slow, or the pupils fail to react to light. A blood glucose test should be performed to exclude hypoglycaemia, plasma calcium concentration estimated, and a lumbar puncture considered to exclude meningitis.

Infants should be nursed in an incubator for easy observation, but if they weigh over 3000 g the thermostat should be turned to the minimum level to prevent overheating.

This type of haemorrhage due to traumatic delivery is now rare. The prognosis is poor. Cranial ultrasound scan may be normal and CT brain scan is the best test to confirm the presence of intracranial haemorrhage.

Other conditions

The cause of sternomastoid 'tumour' is unknown. It is assumed to be related to birth trauma, but it is not usually noticeable at birth. It usually presents after the first week of life. A firm mass, 1–2 cm in diameter, is usually found in the middle or lower third of the sternomastoid muscle but it may be anywhere along its length. It will disappear within a year and usually the infant will then be perfectly normal. The mother is taught by a physiotherapist to move the infant's head passively through the whole range of normal movements daily until the lesion resolves. Subconjunctival haemorrhages and petechiae on the head and neck are common and unimportant. But if there are petechiae on the trunk further investigations are indicated.

Subcutaneous fat necrosis produces a firm subcutaneous area at the site of pressure, especially of the obstetric forceps. It may be red and tender. No treatment is needed. If the site is unusual and the swelling not noticed until a few days after birth, the area of necrosis may be confused with a pyogenic abscess. Extensive subcutaneous fat necrosis is associated with perinatal hypoxia, and hypercalcaemia may develop a few weeks later.

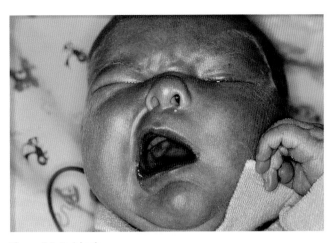

Figure 5.5 Facial palsy.

Pressure on the facial nerve before birth or from obstetric forceps may cause a transient palsy which lasts up to 2 weeks (Figure 5.5). Care of the exposed cornea is essential.

Further reading

Thomas R, Harvey D. (2005) *Paediatrics and Neonatology in Focus.* Elsevier Churchill Livingstone, Edinburgh.

ISBN: 978-1-4051-8037-5

CHAPTER 6

Some Congenital Abnormalities

OVERVIEW

- Many but not all congenital abnormalities can be diagnosed on antenatal ultrasound scanning at around 20 weeks gestation
- Parents should be counselled by fetal medicine specialists, geneticists, neonatal paediatricians and paediatric surgeons to enable them to make informed choices about pregnancy complicated by fetal anomaly

Neural tube defects

A myelomeningocoele is a flat or raised neural plaque partly devoid of skin in the midline over the spine due to abnormal development of the spinal cord and associated deficiency of the dorsal laminae and spines of the vertebrae (Figures 6.1 & 6.2). It is usually found in the lumbosacral region. The absence of the various coverings that normally protect the spinal cord allows meningitis to occur easily. If there are no active movements in the legs and the anus is patulous, the infant will probably be incontinent of urine and faeces for life and never be able to walk unaided. Thoracic lesions and kyphosis are signs of poor prognosis.

Infants with a good prognosis need urgent treatment, so all affected infants should either be seen by a consultant paediatrician without delay or sent to a special centre, where selection for surgery can be made. About 30% of the infants have surgery as a result of this policy. During the first operation the lesion on the back is covered by skin.

Most of these infants develop progressive hydrocephalus later and those considered suitable for surgery require insertion of a ventriculoperitoneal catheter with a valve from a cerebral ventricle to the peritoneal cavity to reduce the cerebrospinal fluid pressure.

Hydrocephalus can be detected by ultrasound examination of the brain. Serial measurements show whether ventricular size is increasing rapidly. In addition, progressive hydrocephalus is confirmed by measuring the circumference of the head at its largest circumference (occipitofrontal) every few days with a disposable paper tape measure, plotting these values on a growth chart, and showing that the head is growing faster than normal.

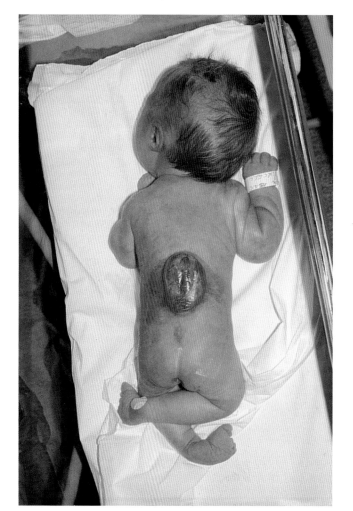

Figure 6.1 Myelomeningocoele.

Raised concentrations of α-fetoprotein are found in the amniotic fluid when the fetus has an open myelomeningocoele or anencephaly. In anencephaly there is absence of the cranial vault and most of the brain.

A routine anomaly scan at around 20 weeks of gestation will detect most neural tube defects and the parents may decide that the pregnancy should be terminated in view of the poor prognosis.

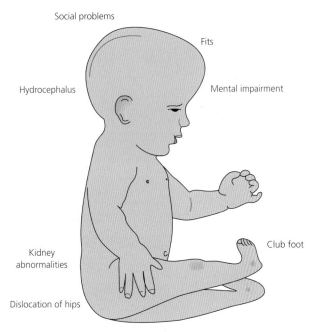

Figure 6.2 Associated features of myelomeningocoele.

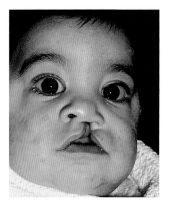

Figure 6.3 Cleft lip and palate.

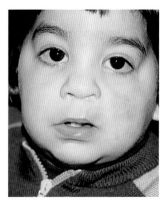

Figure 6.4 Same patient after operation.

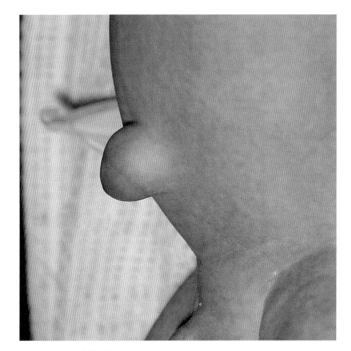

Figure 6.5 Umbilical hernia.

Anencephaly is a lethal condition but some infants survive for a few hours or days after birth.

Microcephaly

The signs of microcephaly are a small head and forehead that is particularly small in relation to the face. The diagnosis is confirmed by showing a small head circumference in relation to the baby's weight and gestational age, and continuing poor growth of the head after birth. It is usually associated with mental impairment. Other congenital abnormalities may be present. Evidence of an intrauterine infection such as toxoplasmosis should be sought and the parents should receive appropriate genetic counselling. The diagnosis may be difficult at birth, but the increasing discrepancy between the head circumference centile and the weight and length centiles with developmental delay clarifies the diagnosis.

Cleft lip and palate

Parents are often severely disturbed by the appearance of these infants and may be reassured by seeing photographs of similar patients before and after their repair operations (Figures 6.3 & 6.4). Cleft lip and cleft palate are often associated. Referral to a specialized multidisciplinary team should be made as soon as possible after birth. A cleft lip, caused by failure of the maxillary process growing towards the midline to fuse with the premaxilla, may be unilateral or bilateral. Minor degrees of cleft palate may be easily missed if the posterior part of the palate is not seen and palpated. Most of these infants feed normally from the breast or bottle. If there are feeding difficulties, a special teat, a large normal teat, a special spade-like spoon, or an ordinary spoon may be tried. The lip is usually repaired at 3 months and the palate before the

age of 1 year. The value of an obturator before operative closure of the palate is controversial. If an obturator is needed, it should be made and fitted within 24 hours of birth. Despite excellent operative results, these children are prone to recurrent otitis media and problems with speech development. Infants born to a family with a parent or sibling with cleft lip and palate, and those born to mothers who have epilepsy, have a higher risk of cleft lip and palate.

Midline abdominal herniae

An umbilical hernia, usually containing omentum and gut, is most common in African infants or West Indians of African descent (Figure 6.5). About 30% of preterm infants who have received mechanical ventilation have an umbilical hernia. No treatment is needed, as the hernia usually disappears spontaneously by the age of 3 years, although in West Indian infants it may take a further 3 years.

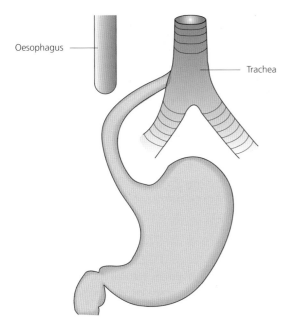

Figure 6.6 Oesophageal atresia with tracheo-oesophageal fistula.

In contrast to an umbilical hernia, the sac of an omphalocoele is covered by peritoneum but incompletely by skin. An omphalocoele is a hernia into the base of the umbilical cord and contains gut and sometimes solid organs like the liver. Immediate transfer to a surgical unit is needed.

Gastroschisis is a more extensive midline abdominal defect which is often associated with chromosomal anomalies such as trisomy 13 or 18. Surgical closure of the defect is indicated if the infant does not have other life-threatening symptoms.

Oesophageal atresia

Oesophageal atresia should be suspected in any newborn baby who has a continual accumulation of frothy secretions in the mouth with drooling, sometimes with cyanotic attacks (Figure 6.6).

The diagnosis of oesophageal atresia is confirmed by attempting to pass a tube down the oesophagus. The tube should have a relatively wide lumen (FG 10), must be stiff enough to prevent coiling in the upper oesophageal pouch, and should have a radio-opaque line so that the position can be checked by a chest radiograph. The tube should be aspirated every few minutes to keep the upper pouch clear until the infant reaches a specialized surgical unit.

Oesophageal atresia will be suspected antenatally if there is polyhydramnios and difficulty in detecting a normal stomach bubble at the routine 18–24 weeks anomaly scan.

Oesophageal atresia may be associated with a tracheal fistula (Figure 6.6).

Multiple abnormalities

Infants with multiple abnormalities should be examined and investigated by a paediatrician without delay to ensure correct management and to provide the information needed for genetic

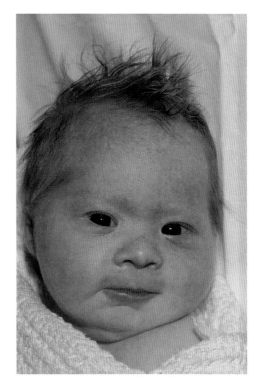

Figure 6.7 Down syndrome.

counselling. Some of the infants may have a recognizable syndrome and investigations may show a chromosomal defect or evidence of intrauterine infection.

The most common presentation is the infant with possible Down syndrome (trisomy 21). Although a scoring system for a large number of clinical features has been used in the past, any infant with suspected Down syndrome should have a blood chromosome analysis performed.

The most useful features suggesting the diagnosis are the flattened facial appearance with palpebral fissures that slant upwards and outwards, prominent epicanthic folds, baggy cheeks and white spots on the iris (Brushfield spots) (Figure 6.7). A flat occiput, poor limb tone and single palmar crease are suggestive but not specific signs. About 2% of normal infants have a single palmar crease in one hand, and prominent epicanthic folds are even more common. Congenital heart disease, most commonly an atrioventricular septal defect, occur in approximately 30% of infants with Down syndrome and will be detected by performing an echocardiogram, as a definite murmur may not be present until several weeks after birth. All infants with Down syndrome have developmental delay and slow growth. Parents find it helpful to meet with the multidisciplinary team who will monitor their infant's progress at an early stage. Advice about helping their infant to learn and progress is provided by skilled paediatric therapists.

Further reading

Thomas R, Harvey D. (2005) *Paediatrics and Neonatology in Focus.* Elsevier Churchill Livingstone, Edinburgh.

CHAPTER 7

Routine Examination of the Newborn

OVERVIEW

- The main purpose of the routine neonatal examination within the first 48 hours of birth is to confirm normality

- A trained clinician will be able diagnose abnormalities of the eyes, heart and hips. Mothers look very closely at their newborn infants and will notice most of the other external congenital anomalies and normal variants

- Routine screening for phenylketonuria, hypothyroidism, cystic fibrosis and sickle cell disease is carried out between 5 and 7 days after birth

- All newborn infants have a neonatal audiological screening test within a few days after birth or just before discharge home if they are born prematurely (page 15)

Immediately after birth all infants should be examined to exclude gross congenital abnormalities or evidence of birth trauma. Later, preferably within 24 hours of birth or on the morning after delivery, every infant should be examined again in detail (Box 7.1). Early examination of the heart and hips will reveal physiological cardiac bruits and ligamentous clicks which disappear within hours of birth. They are of no clinical significance, but generate anxiety for the parents and the infant will require repeat examination the next day. The obstetric notes should be checked to determine whether the infant has been at special risk – for example, from maternal ill-health or a difficult delivery. A systematic approach should be used so that abnormalities are not missed. The infant must be completely undressed and in a good light. The mother should be present during the examination so that the results of the examination can be discussed with her and so that she can voice her anxieties. Minor common normal variations of normality can cause great anxiety to a new parent and reassurance from an experienced doctor or midwife is always helpful.

Skin

Diffuse capillary naevi on the face, eyelids, or occiput (often called stork bite marks) are common and resolve within a few months. Milia are pinpoint white spots on the face which resolve spontaneously. See Box 7.2.

The 'strawberry mark' starts as a tiny red spot and grows rapidly for several weeks until it has a raised red appearance with small white areas, suggesting the seeds of a strawberry (Figure 7.1). Such marks are common in preterm babies. They may occur anywhere on the body but cause no symptoms, except on the eyelids, where

Box 7.2 **Common skin findings**

- Capillary naevi – stork bite marks
- Strawberry naevi
- Milia
- Erythema toxicum

Box 7.1 **Routine neonatal examination**

- Eyes – red reflex
- Heart – no murmurs and normal femoral pulses
- Hips – no instability or dislocation
- Anus patent
- Normal external genitalia
- Testes descended

ABC of the First Year, Sixth edition. By B. Valman and R. Thomas. © 2009 Blackwell Publishing, ISBN: 978-1-4051-8037-5.

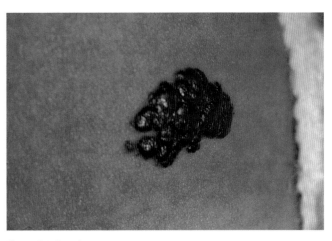

Figure 7.1 Strawberry naevus.

they may prevent easy opening of the eyes and need treatment to preserve normal vision. Strawberry naevi grow, often rapidly, for 3–9 months, but at least 90% resolve spontaneously, either completely or partially. Resolution usually begins at 6–12 months and is complete in half the children by the age of 5 and in 70% by the age of 7 years. In 80% of cases these naevi resolve completely without trace.

The port wine stain is not raised and may be extensive (Figure 7.2). It does not resolve, but the skin texture remains normal. When the naevus occurs in the distribution of the trigeminal nerve, there may be an associated intracranial vascular anomaly.

Neonatal erythema (erythema 'toxicum') consists of blotchy ill-defined areas of bright erythema surrounding white or yellow wheals which may resemble septic spots (Figure 7.3). Neonatal erythema toxicum usually appears on the second day of life and in most infants clears within 48 hours. The lesions contain many eosinophils and have no pathological importance. Neonatal erythema is more common in full-term infants. By ringing individual lesions with a skin pencil they can be shown to disappear in a few hours, to be replaced by others elsewhere. This contrasts with septic lesions, which appear later and do not resolve so quickly.

Mongolian blue spots are patchy accumulations of pigment, especially over the buttocks and lower back in infants of races with pigmented skins. They are common in babies of African or Mongolian descent, but also occur in Italian and Greek babies. They may be mistaken for bruises by inexperienced observers and a wrong diagnosis of non-accidental injury made. They become less obvious as the skin darkens.

A midline pit over the spine is most commonly found over the coccyx, where it does not usually communicate with the spinal canal. A midline pit anywhere else along the spine may be connected with an underlying sinus, which may communicate with the spinal canal and requires excision to prevent the entry of bacteria and meningitis. An ultrasound scan of the lower back and spine will show if there is a fistulous connection to the spinal canal.

Head and neck

An infant with the Pierre Robin syndrome has a small lower jaw, glossoptosis and cleft palate (Figure 7.4). The infant must be nursed prone to prevent the tongue falling backwards and occluding the airway. A small jaw (micrognathia) may occur alone or with other abnormalities. As the child grows the small size of the lower jaw becomes less obvious.

Nodules of epithelial cells resembling pearls (Epstein's pearls) just lateral to the midline on the hard palate are a normal finding. A cluster of these pearls may be present at the junction of the hard and soft palates and occasionally on the foreskin.

Heart murmurs

In the first 2 days of life one of the most common findings is an infant who is feeding normally, but who is found to have a short systolic murmur during a routine examination. The murmur is usually due to a patent ductus arteriosus and has usually disappeared by the time the infant is examined again a few days later. An electrocardiogram (ECG) or chest radiograph is unnecessary.

If a long murmur is first heard around the eighth day of life, a chest radiograph, ECG and echocardiogram should be performed and the infant seen by a paediatrician or paediatric cardiologist. Most of these murmurs are due to a ventricular septal defect (VSD) or mild pulmonary stenosis with no symptoms (Figure 7.5).

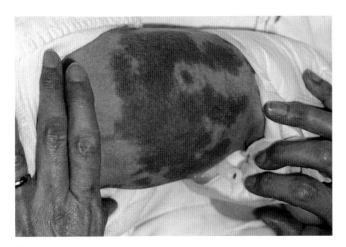

Figure 7.2 Port wine stain.

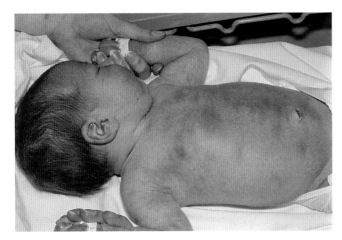

Figure 7.3 Neonatal erythema.

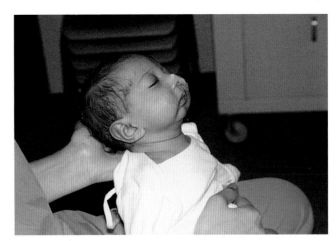

Figure 7.4 Pierre Robin syndrome.

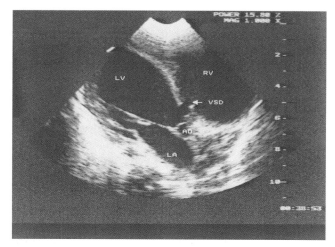

Figure 7.5 Echocardiogram showing ventricular septal defect (VSD).

Most VSDs close spontaneously before the infant reaches the age of 5 years.

The normal respiratory rate at rest is less than 60/min and there should be no recession of the chest wall or below the mandible. If there is any murmur and the infant is feeding poorly or has a respiratory rate faster than 60/min at rest, a chest radiograph and ECG should be performed and the baby seen by a paediatrician urgently. These symptoms and signs may indicate congestive heart failure usually due to multiple heart defects.

Cyanosis of the hands and feet is common in newborn infants and has no importance if the tongue is of normal colour and the infant is feeding normally.

Abdomen

The liver edge is normally 1–2 cm below the costal margin in the midclavicular line. In a thin, relaxed infant the kidneys may be palpable bimanually.

The inguinal areas are inspected for the presence of a hernia. Absence of the femoral pulses suggests that coarctation of the aorta is present. The blood pressure is measured in all four limbs and referral to a cardiologist is made.

Failure to pass urine in the first 36 hours or a poor urinary stream suggests posterior urethral valves in a boy. An enlarged bladder may be palpable. Diagnosis is confirmed by an ultrasound examination, which may show hydronephrosis, and cystourethrogram to confirm the outflow tract obstruction (Figure 7.6).

Patency of the anus is confirmed by inspection.

Genitalia

The prepuce or foreskin is attached to the penis at birth and no attempt should be made to retract it.

A hooded prepuce suggests hypospadias with the urethral orifice at the base of the glans penis (Figure 7.7). If the urethral meatus is adequate, no immediate treatment is needed, but the infant must not be circumcised and should be referred to a paediatric urologist.

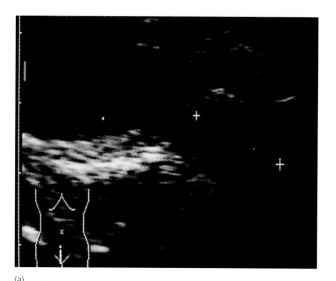

(a)

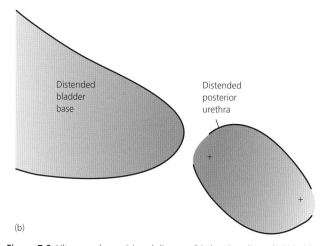

(b)

Figure 7.6 Ultrasound scan (a) and diagram (b) showing distended bladder and distended posterior urethra due to urethral valves.

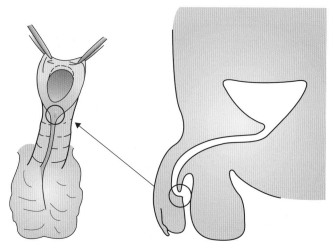

Figure 7.7 Hypospadias.

If the urethral orifice is nearer the perineum, the adrenogenital syndrome should be considered. In the adrenogenital syndrome cortisol secretion fails and the adrenals produce excessive androgen. Girls become virilized, with enlargement of the clitoris and fusion of the labia, and may be mistaken for boys (see page 60). In boys the genitalia are normal at birth.

Intersex is a less common cause of ambiguity of the external genitalia and a paediatrician should be consulted without delay. An accurate diagnosis is an emotional and social emergency. The parents should be advised that the baby should not be named until the results of chromosome studies are available.

Small hydrocoeles usually disappear spontaneously during the first month, but an associated inguinal hernia should be excluded.

Poor development of the scrotum suggests that an undescended testis is present. Undescended testis is especially common in preterm infants, in whom the testes usually descend during the first 3 months after birth. An undescended testis is present in 30% of preterm and 3% of term infants at birth. An infant with an undescended testis should be seen again at the age of 3 months. At that time 5% of preterm infants and 1% of term babies will still have an undescended testis and they should be referred for surgery, which is performed at about the age of 2 years. If the baby develops an associated hernia, the operation will be needed as a relative emergency.

As the cremasteric reflex is usually absent at birth, the testis cannot be retractile. If there is any doubt about whether a testis is descended the examiner should (a) palpate the pubic tubercle with one hand, (b) hold the testis between the thumb and forefinger of the other hand and gently draw it down to its fullest extent and then (c) measure the distance from the pubic tubercle to the centre of the firm globular testis (Figure 7.8). At term the testis, if fully descended, lies 4–7 cm from the tubercle. If the distance is under 4 cm the testis has not completely descended. In preterm babies, who are more likely to have undescended testes and whose testes are smaller, 2.5 cm has been arbitrarily chosen to divide descent from non-descent.

Spontaneous primary descent of the testes rarely occurs after the age of 4 months and never after 1 year. After the neonatal period an active cremasteric reflex can easily pull the testis out of the scrotum, especially if the examiner's hands are cold. The mother will often have noted whether the testes are both in the scrotum after a warm bath, and a retractile testis will descend into the scrotum when the thigh and knee are maximally flexed on that side (Figure 7.9).

In girls a small amount of vaginal bleeding is common, usually 5–7 days after birth, and follows withdrawal of maternal or placental oestrogens, which are transmitted to the fetus before birth. White vaginal discharge, a mucousy posterior hymenal tag or prolapse of the vaginal mucosa are normal (Figure 7.10).

In either sex physiological enlargement of the breasts may occur towards the end of the first week. This enlargement, which may be unilateral, resolves within a few weeks, but if there is local redness, a breast abscess should be suspected.

Circumcision

In 95% of babies the foreskin and glans of the penis are still united at birth. It has been found that the foreskin can be retracted by the age of 1 year in about half the babies and by the age of 3 years in nine out of ten. No attempt should be made to

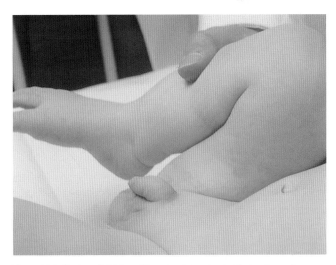

Figure 7.9 Flexion of thigh and knee to determine testicular descent.

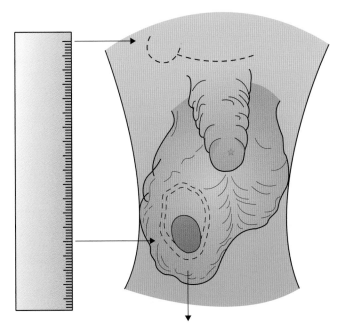

Figure 7.8 Measurement of testicular descent.

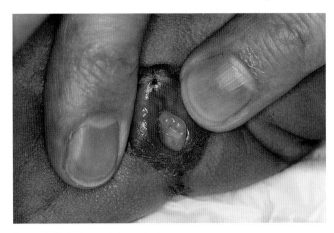

Figure 7.10 Prolapse of the vaginal mucosa.

retract the foreskin until the baby is about 4 years old. Attempts to retract the foreskin earlier are likely to injure the mucosa, causing bleeding followed by adhesions, and circumcision may later become necessary. Parents often request circumcision to be carried out because the prepucial orifice appears small. In most cases the adequacy of the orifice can be shown by gently stretching the foreskin distally (Figure 7.11) and no attempt should be made to retract the foreskin. Before the age of 4 years the only medical indications for circumcision are recurrent purulent balanitis and ballooning of the foreskin at the beginning of micturition.

Most circumcisions are performed as a religious ritual, in Jewish boys on the eighth day of life and in Muslim boys between the ages of 3 and 15 years. If circumcision is performed, the infant will need appropriate analgesia or a brief anaesthetic.

Club foot and extra digits

Muscular imbalance due to the posture of the infant's feet *in utero* is the commonest cause of club foot. In postural club foot it should be possible to dorsiflex the foot fully and to obtain passive inversion to 90° (Figure 7.12). The mother should be taught to manipulate the foot through the whole range of movements after each feed for several days after birth, although the shape usually reverts to normal within a few weeks even without treatment. In contrast, in structural club foot the range of passive movements is restricted and orthopaedic advice on strapping, manipulation or serial plasters is needed as soon as possible after birth.

To detect extra digits, the digits should be counted with the infant's palms open, or an extra thumb may be missed (Figure 7.13). Polydactyly requires the advice of a plastic surgeon to determine which digit should be removed at the age of 3–4 years for the best functional results. Extra fingers and toes are often familial and vary from an apparently normal digit to a skin tag. The latter can be carefully tied off at the narrow base with a sterile silk thread and will separate by aseptic necrosis.

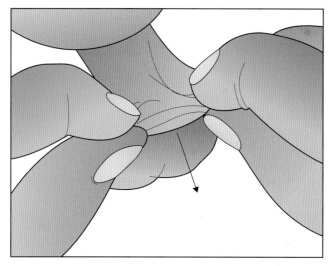

Figure 7.11 Stretching foreskin distally.

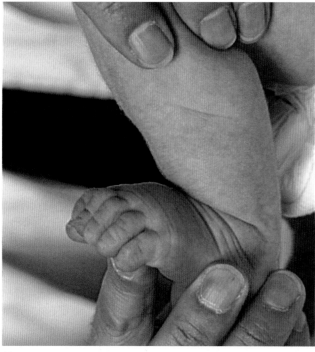

(a)

(b)

Figure 7.12 (a) Postural talipes. (b) Structural talipes.

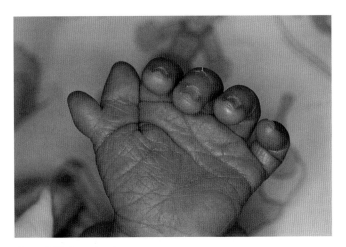

Figure 7.13 Extra thumb.

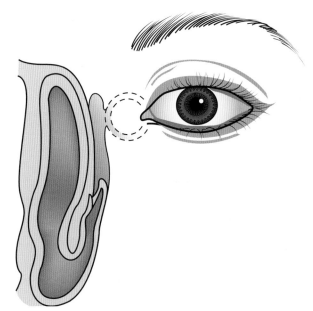

Figure 7.15 Tear duct.

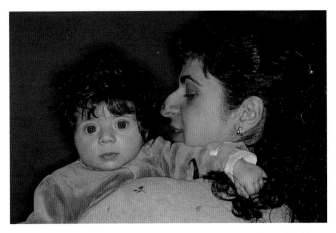

Figure 7.14 Eyes open when the infant is held over the mother's shoulder.

Central nervous system and eyes

To assess the central nervous system the alertness of the infant and the symmetry of spontaneous movements should be noted. The tension of the anterior fontanelle and the width of the fontanelle should be palpated while the infant is at rest and the head circumference should be measured. A more detailed neurological examination is not required unless there is a special indication.

Babies will open their eyes when being fed or when held upright over someone's shoulder (Figure 7.14). Babies will follow the movements of an examiner's face provided that the distance is 50 cm or more. The pupils of every baby should be examined with an ophthalmoscope at a distance of 50 cm. A bright red glow is seen, which is a reflection of light from the back of the retina. Absence of this 'red reflex' is found in congenital cataract, which produces a dull grey appearance.

Watering eye

If there is persistent watering of the eye with clear fluid, the tear duct is probably blocked (Figure 7.15). No action is required until at least the age of 1 year, when the infant can be referred to an ophthalmic surgeon.

Rarely, the tear duct is probed, but most ophthalmic surgeons prefer to take no action because the condition resolves spontaneously in most infants and probing may induce fibrosis of the tear duct. If there is repeated or persistent purulent discharge, the possibility of chlamydia infection should be considered and arrangements made with the laboratory for specimens to be taken. Chlamydia opthalmitis requires systemic antibiotics in order to prevent recurrence.

Taking blood

Capillary blood taken from infants aged up to 2 years can be used for a variety of tests. The commonest is the Guthrie test, but capillary blood may also be used for blood glucose testing, haemoglobin estimations and most biochemical tests.

The best site for taking capillary blood from an infant aged under 6 months is the heel. In older infants the thumb is a better site. The heel must be warm. If it is cold, the infant's foot should be dipped into hand-hot water (40°C) for 5 minutes and dried thoroughly. The examiner then holds the infant's foot by encircling the ball of the heel with thumb and forefinger (Figure 7.16). The site selected for the heel prick must be on the side of the heel; if the ball or back of the heel is used a painful ulcer may form (Figure 7.17).

The site is wiped with isopropyl alcohol and allowed to dry. A spring-loaded lancet introducer is used.

The initial drop of blood should be wiped away with a dry cotton swab and succeeding drops allowed to drip into the container, onto the Guthrie test card or onto the end of a glucometer strip. To milk blood into the heel the examiner should squeeze gently and release the fingers around the infant's calf and keep the heel below the rest of the leg. Up to 2 mL of blood can be obtained, but the sample should be taken carefully, avoiding excessive force when squeezing, in order to prevent haemolysis of the blood which may give inaccurate results. When the required volume has been obtained, the heel is wiped and the wound pressed with a clean cotton wool ball. A small plaster should then be applied.

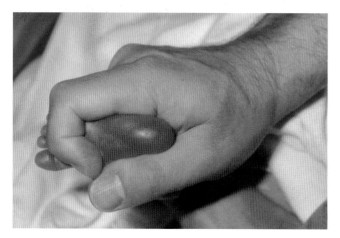

Figure 7.16 Holding foot for taking blood.

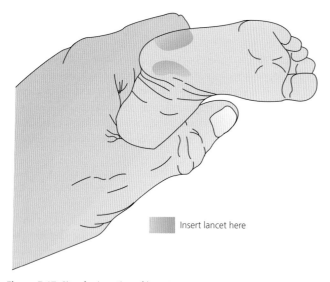

Insert lancet here

Figure 7.17 Sites for insertion of lancet.

Routine blood spot screening (Box 7.3)

The Guthrie test detects high blood concentrations of phenylalanine, which indicate that the infant probably has phenylketonuria. Drops of blood are taken by heel prick after 5–7 days' breast or bottle feeding. and placed on the special absorbent card provided (Figure 7.18). The blood is usually taken by the midwife if the infant is at home. If the test is positive, the infant should be admitted to hospital to confirm the diagnosis, as he or she may need a special low phenylalanine diet to prevent brain damage.

Some laboratories use the plasma thyroid-stimulating hormone and others the plasma thyroxine value as the screening test for hypothyroidism. An elevated plasma immunoreactive trypsin level in the newborn period is suggestive of cystic fibrosis and definitive gene testing and a sweat test will be needed to confirm the diagnosis. The screening blood card with four spots is used for the Guthrie test, the tests for hypothyroidism and cystic fibrosis. In some populations with a high prevalence of sickle cell disease, routine haemoglobin electrophoresis is done on a separate blood spot on the first day of life.

Talking to parents

Whenever possible both parents should be seen together (Figure 7.19). If an abnormality is found during the routine examination, some indication must be given to the mother so that arrangements can be made to see both parents. Particularly if the problem is likely to be long term, the doctor who will continue the long-term care should speak to the parents initially. Ideally, a nurse should be present as well, since the parents will probably ask all the questions again as soon as the doctor has left.

The diagnosis should be explained in terms that the parents can understand and the positive aspects should be emphasized.

Box 7.3 **Routine blood spot screening can detect:**

- phenylketonuria
- hypothyroidism
- cystic fibrosis
- sickle cell disease

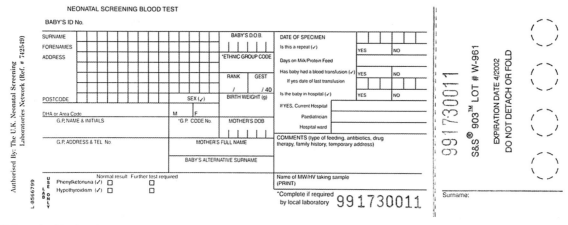

Figure 7.18 Screening blood card.

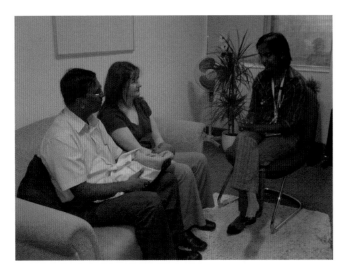

Figure 7.19 Talking to parents.

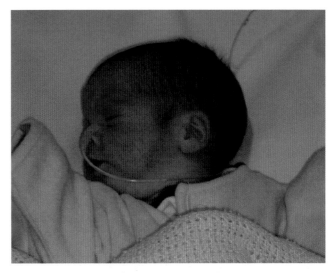

Figure 7.20 Position for sleeping.

For example, if the probable diagnosis is ventricular septal defect, it is not necessary to explain that there is a remote possibility of multiple cardiac defects. After a difficult forceps delivery, it is better to say that most babies develop normally rather than say they may be slightly disabled. An unnecessarily pessimistic prognosis based on out-of-date information may alter a mother's attitude towards her baby and impair her attachment to him or her.

In discussing management, the help and support that will be given by social workers or therapists should be emphasized and the parents advised to tell their relations and friends the diagnosis rather than hide it.

A doctor with only limited experience of a particular problem should tell the parents that he or she needs to seek further advice rather than guess at the answer. Parents often cling to the first opinion and may find it difficult to accept a more experienced view later. A statement of the facts – for example, that there is an abnormality of the spine – may be given with the assurance that a more experienced doctor will have a discussion with them later.

Useful advice for new parents

Sleeping position of infants

It is recommended that babies should be placed on their back to sleep as this has been shown to reduce the risk of cot death (Figure 7.20). Healthy babies placed on their backs are not more likely to choke if they vomit. The mattress used in a baby's cot should be firm, flat and clean, and covered in waterproof material. Pillows should not be used. To prevent the baby wriggling down under the covers, a baby's feet should be placed at the foot of the cot or pram (Figure 7.21). There has been an increase in flattening of the head predominantly on one side (plagiocephaly) or the occiput (brachycephaly) and delay in achieving head control when pulled from the supine to upright position in recent years, probably associated with back sleeping in the early months. Mothers should be encouraged to place their infant in the supine position when it is safe to do so when they are awake and during periods of play. Flattening of the head and delay in head control improve with increasing age and do

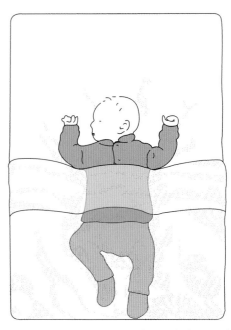

Figure 7.21 Correct sleeping position, with feet at the bottom of the cot.

not require any special intervention. Although the use of helmets is advocated by some authorities, they are expensive, inconvenient and unsightly as they are supposed to be worn 23 hours a day until 1 year of age, and they are of unproven benefit.

By 6–7 months of age, many babies will roll over onto their front during sleep. There is no need for concern about this, as the risk of cot death is markedly reduced by this age. There are, however, certain circumstances in which babies should be nursed on their side or prone (on their front). These include some babies in neonatal units, babies with severe gastro-oesophageal reflux, babies receiving treatment in splints for unstable hips and babies with Pierre Robin syndrome.

Cellular blankets are ideal and duvets or loose bedding should be avoided. An infant should not sleep on a sofa or bed with a

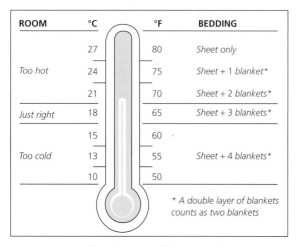

ROOM	°C	°F	BEDDING
	27	80	*Sheet only*
Too hot	24	75	*Sheet + 1 blanket**
	21	70	*Sheet + 2 blankets**
Just right	18	65	*Sheet + 3 blankets**
	15	60	
Too cold	13	55	*Sheet + 4 blankets**
	10	50	

* A double layer of blankets counts as two blankets

Figure 7.22 Amount of bedding required for a range of room temperatures to keep the infant's temperature at the optimum level.

parent as overlaying may occur. It has been recommended that the infant should sleep in the same room as the parent for the first 6 months of life.

Avoiding smoking near babies

Smoking in pregnancy by the mother will reduce the birthweight of the infant by approximately 200 g at term and increases the risk of cot death. Babies exposed to cigarette smoke after birth are more likely to suffer wheezing and respiratory infections. It is best if everyone, especially parents, refrains from smoking in the same house or room as a baby.

Temperature

Overheating a baby may increase the risk of cot death. A room temperature of about 18°C (65°F) is comfortable for babies as well as adults (Figure 7.22).

Car seats

Whenever a baby is taken in a car, they should always be strapped into a baby seat or rear-facing infant carrier. In the UK there is a legal requirement for all children under the age of 12 years to be in an age- and size-appropriate car seat with suitable safety restraints. It is not safe to nurse a baby on the lap in a car, even if the adult is wearing a seat belt.

Foreign travel with infants

Families are more mobile and are increasingly seeking advice about air travel with young children. Infants are at increased risk of experiencing earache during take-off and landing because the drainage of their Eustachian tubes may be partially blocked with fluid and mucus. Feeding the infant may help by producing a partial Valsalva manoeuvre, but may not be possible because of safety restrictions in the aircraft.

Travel to foreign countries is best avoided until the completion of the routine infant immunizations after 4 months of age. BCG should also be given if travelling to a country with a high prevalence of tuberculosis.

If travelling to a country where malaria is endemic, antimalarial prophylaxis is essential for young infants and can be safely given to all infants, provided that they do not have neonatal jaundice. The same drugs as are prescribed for adults can be used in appropriate dosage for infants:

- first month of life: one-eighth adult dose
- 1 month to 1 year of age: one-quarter adult dose.

Boiled or bottled water should be used for drinking water and preparation of infant formula feeds abroad. Parents should be advised not to use commercially produced mineral water with a sodium content more than 20 mg/L, as a high salt intake can be harmful in young infants. Changes in drinking water and diet may cause an alteration in intestinal flora and diarrhoea in young infants. Meticulous attention to hygiene will help to prevent gastroenteritis. It is advisable to carry sachets of powdered oral infant rehydration mixture when travelling abroad with young infants, as they may not be readily available in some countries.

The skin of young infants is very susceptible to sunburn and must always be protected with liberal applications of high-factor sunblock, hats, and sun shields or umbrellas in hot sunny climates.

Cot deaths

About one baby in every 2000 born alive dies suddenly and unexpectedly between the ages of 1 week and 2 years. Typically, an apparently healthy baby (or occasionally one with only minor symptoms) is put in a cot to rest and some time later is found dead. Although an infant may be face down in the cot with the bedclothes over him or her, suffocation should not be assumed. Sometimes vomit, which may be blood tinged, is found around the mouth or on the bedding, but regurgitation usually occurs after death and is not the cause of death.

In some cases autopsy discloses an unsuspected congenital abnormality or rapidly fatal infection. But usually there is no evidence of severe disease, though there might be slight reddening of the tracheal mucosa.

Parents often blame themselves and may worry that the infant suffocated as a result of neglect. They should be told that their feelings of guilt are a natural reaction and the doctor should explain to them, and to anyone who was looking after the baby when death occurred, that cot death is a well recognized, but poorly understood condition and that no one is to blame for the infant's death. See Boxes 7.4 and 7.5.

Parents must also be told that because the death is of unknown cause the coroner will have to be told as a matter of routine and that there will be an autopsy examination. If the parents want to see the infant's body (and they should be asked), the infant is clothed and a doctor or nurse should be present to answer questions and provide

---

Box 7.4 **Foundation for the Study of Infant Deaths (FSID)**

Artillery House, 11–19 Artillery Row, London SW1 IRT
General enquiries telephone: 020 7222 8001; 24-hour
helpline: 020 7233 2090; www.sids.org.uk

Birth details

Date of birth _____ / _____ / _____
Time of birth _____
Weeks of pregnancy _____
Method of delivery _____
Place of birth _____
Problems during pregnancy or birth:
(1) _____
(2) _____
(3) _____
(4) _____

Meconium passed within 24 hr   Yes/No
In special care baby unit   Yes/No
Any neonatal contraindication
to immunisation   Yes/No
Risk factors for congenital
dislocation of hip   Yes/No
Risk factors for hearing
loss   Yes/No/Not Known
Feeding at discharge   Breast/bottle/both

Blood tests done

Phenylketonuria	Yes/No	Norm/Abn
Thyroid test	Yes/No	Norm/Abn
Haemoglobinopathies	Yes/No	Norm/Abn
Cystic fibrosis	Yes/No	Norm/Abn
Hearing test	Yes/No	Norm/Abn
BCG	Yes/No	

Please use ball point pen and press firmly

Infant Hospital NO. _____
Birth Wt. _____ kg   Head circ. _____ cm
Apgar at 1 & 5 mins _____
(Tick box if examination done and write in
'comments' if problem)

		Comments
Skull sutures	☐	_____
Skin	☐	_____
Eyes – red reflex	☐	_____
Palate	☐	_____
Heart	☐	_____
Abdomen	☐	_____
Genitalia	☐	_____
Hips	☐	_____
Limbs/spine	☐	_____

Significant abnormality or condition _____
_____
_____

Follow-up hospital appointment   Yes/No
Reason/details _____
_____
_____

Birth details

Immunisations

ALL CHILDREN SHOULD RECEIVE IMMUNISATIONS except a very few children who:
1. are suffering from a feverish illness – when the immunisation should be postponed until full recovery.
2. have had a severe reaction to a previous immunisation.
3. have an illness or are taking medicines that interfere with their ability to fight infections.

CHILDREN TAKING ANTIBIOTICS CAN BE IMMUNISED.
Before each immunisation the doctor or nurse will make sure that it is all right to give your child the vaccine.

Further comments on consultation sheets: YES/NO

Please use ball point pen and press firmly.

Age due	Site of injection	Vaccine	Date given						Batch number	Signature in full	Treatment centre code
8 weeks	RL/LL.... RL/LL....	DTaP/IPV/HiB PCV									
12 weeks	RL/LL.... RL/LL....	DTaP/IPV/HiB Men C									
16 weeks	RL/LL.... RL/LL....	DTaP/IPV/HiB Men C PCV									
12 months		Hib/Men C									
13 months		MMR (1st dose) PCV									

Immunisations

Figure 7.23 Routine examination of newborn and immunisations.

Box 7.5 **Prevention of sudden infant death**

Although sudden infant death is very rare, it is important to follow the latest guidelines for prevention. These are:
- put your baby to sleep on his or her back
- do not smoke; keep your baby out of smoky atmospheres
- do not let your baby get too warm
- put your baby at the foot of the cot so that he or she cannot wriggle under the covers
- contact your doctor if you think your baby is unwell

support. Parents should be encouraged to see the infant's body as this will help the grieving process. Discussion with the parents will determine who is best to help with their grieving.

The family doctor and health visitor should be informed of the death immediately. The family doctor should explain the results of the autopsy to the parents or arrange for a paediatrician to do this.

Brothers and sisters of the infant who has died will need reassurance that they will not die and are in a safe and loving environment. The concept of the finality of death may not be attained until the age of 8 years. Children may be disturbed by the emotional distress of the parents and this may cause behavioural or sleep problems.

Further reading

Personal Child Health Record (Red Book) given to all parents by midwife or health visitor (Figure 7.23).

CHAPTER 8

Dislocated and Dislocatable Hip in the Newborn

OVERVIEW

- Clinical testing for stability of the hips is an important part of the routine neonatal examination which is best done at around 24 hours of age. However, a small number of infants have clinically normal hips at birth and present with late dislocation

- Infants at high risk of developmental dysplasia and dislocation should have an ultrasound scan at 4–6 weeks of age and if this is abnormal they should be referred to a paediatric orthopaedic surgeon for ongoing management

Congenital dislocated hip and dislocatable hip are probably the most important asymptomatic congenital abnormalities to detect, as early treatment is simple and usually effective. In the first 12 hours of life 10 per 1000 infants in the UK have a hip abnormality. When the examination is carried out 24–36 hours after birth, the incidence of hip abnormality falls to about 7 per 1000 births. Formerly, when they were all left untreated in the newborn, the incidence of established dislocated hip was 1 in 800 children. There may be a family history of the condition; the anomaly is more common in girls and after the extended breech position *in utero* (Box 8.1). There is a higher incidence in some countries, such as Italy and the former Yugoslavia.

The best time to examine the infant's hips is between 24 and 36 hours after birth, as the tendency to provoke regurgitation is less and there is less ligamentous laxity by that time. The examiner's hands should be warm and the infant should be placed on their back with the sheet spread completely flat. The infant should be fully relaxed and this may be encouraged by putting an empty sterile feeding teat in their mouth if necessary. The gentle abduction

Box 8.1 **Special risk of congenital dislocated hip**

- Born in breech position
- Family history of congenital dislocated hip
- Foot deformity e.g. talipes equino varus
- Myelomeningocoele

ABC of the First Year, Sixth edition. By B. Valman and R. Thomas. © 2009 Blackwell Publishing, ISBN: 978-1-4051-8037-5.

test, followed by Barlow's test, should be carried out in all cases. Unnecessary trauma to the delicate hip joint and its capsule must be avoided.

Gentle abduction test

The gentle abduction test will detect hips that are in the dislocated position at rest. Each hip should be examined separately, while the opposite thigh is gently fixed by the examiner's other hand. Both the knee and the hip should be flexed to a right angle and the knee held so that the examiner's thumb is parallel to the medial aspect of the lower thigh, while the middle two fingers lie along the whole length of the lateral aspect of the femur (Figures 8.1 & 8.2). The tips of the examiner's fingers thus lie over the greater trochanter.

The thigh should be held *lightly* and neither pushed down towards the cot surface nor pulled up towards the examiner's

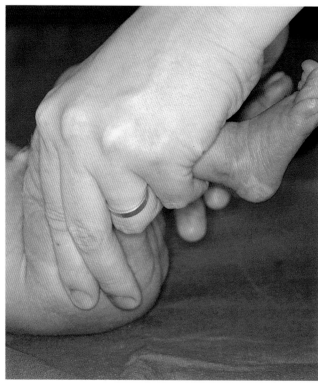

Figure 8.1 Gentle abduction test showing position of examiner's fingers.

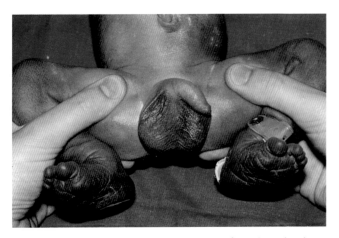

Figure 8.2 Gentle abduction test showing position of examiner's thumb.

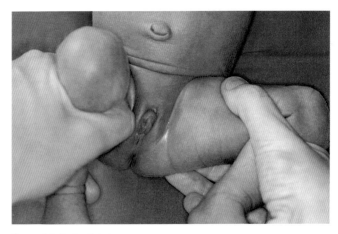

Figure 8.3 Barlow's test.

face. It should then be allowed to abduct very gently and slowly by the weight of the infant's leg until abduction is complete. The thigh should never be forcibly abducted and it is unnecessary to obtain abduction beyond 10° above the flat. While abducting the thigh, the examiner may feel or see the head of the femur slip, jerk or jolt forward into the acetabulum. A temporary interruption in the flow of abduction at a point about midway through abduction precedes the sensation of this abnormal movement of the head of the femur.

If the joint capsule is very lax, the reduction jolt may be missed unless great care is taken.

Barlow's test

The object of Barlow's test is to identify dislocatable hips in which the head of the femur can be gently jolted posteriorly over the posterior lip of the acetabular labrum to lie temporarily out of the acetabulum and those dislocated hips in which the head of the femur can be jolted forwards to lie temporarily in the acetabulum.

Each hip should again be examined separately while the opposite thigh is gently fixed by the examiner's other hand. The infant's hip should be flexed to a right angle and the knee more acutely flexed. The examiner should place a thumb as high as possible on the medial aspect of the upper femur while the tips of the middle two fingers grasp the greater trochanter laterally (Figure 8.3).

The thigh is held lightly in a position of only minimal abduction and then an attempt is made to push the femoral head gently posteriorly and slightly superiorly, while at the same time the examiner's hand is internally rotated through not more than 25°. This is followed by reversing the whole movement. No excessive force is used and only a very limited range of movement employed in the test.

The movement of the head of the femur out and in, or in and out, of the acetabulum produces a jolting or jerking movement, *which can be seen and felt by the examiner. It cannot be heard by an individual with average hearing.* The sensation is like that of a gear lever engaging.

Hips that show excessive movement of the head of the femur within the joint, without being actually dislocatable, are classified as normal.

Ligamentous laxity. In at least 10% of infants this examination evokes a noise, click, snap or grating sensation, but there is no abnormal movement of the femoral head. Such hips should be considered normal and no follow-up is required. Because of confusion about its meaning, the term 'clicking hip' should be abandoned.

Examination of the hips should be performed more than 24 hours after birth because fewer ligamentous clicks will be found.

Ultrasound in screening

If ultrasound screening is undertaken in every infant before leaving hospital, imaging facilities will be required 7 days a week. Twenty per cent of hips may be considered abnormal and the majority will resolve to normal within 4 weeks (Figures 8.4 & 8.5).

Selective screening with ultrasound of infants with a clinical hip abnormality or risk factors for congenital dislocated hip (breech delivery, positive family history or foot deformity) reduces the screened population and allows treatment options to be delayed and targeted effectively. A 2002 study showed that this approach has not reduced the prevalence of late cases of congenital dislocated hip and it has been suggested that selective ultrasound screening is dependent upon more vigorous clinical screening and careful selection of risk factors.

Ultrasound in diagnosis and management

Shallow acetabulae occur with normal hips and delaying ultrasound screening examination to 4–6 weeks in clinically stable hips will allow treatment to be targeted to those hips that require splintage and thus reduce treatment rates without compromising the results of this treatment.

Weekly ultrasound studies can be used to confirm hip relocation and treatment progress while the infant is in a malleable splint or Pavlik harness. Sonographic evidence of continuing femoral head

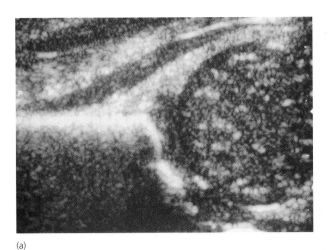

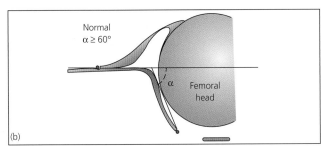

Figure 8.4 (a) Ultrasound of normal hip; (b) diagram.

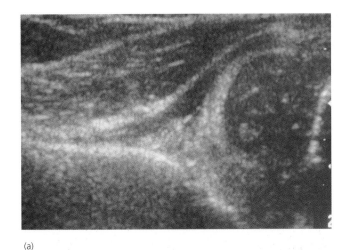

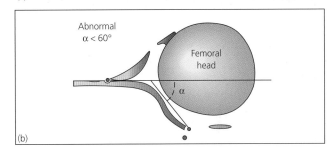

Figure 8.5 (a) Ultrasound of abnormal hip; (b) diagram.

dislocation, despite splintage, allows treatment to be abandoned and thus the risk of avascular necrosis is reduced. The appearance of the ossific nucleus in the cartilaginous femoral head (usually delayed in congenital dislocated hip) is identified sonographically several weeks before it is visualized radiologically.

Recommended screening

Infants born after a vertex presentation who have normal hips on clinical examination and do not have any risk factors will continue to receive clinical screening using the neonatal examination. Infants who are judged to be at risk of congenital dislocated hip because they:
- were born in breech position or
- have a family history of congenital dislocated hip or
- have a foot deformity

should have an ultrasound scan at 4–6 weeks of age, in addition to the clinical screening tests. If they are clinically normal and the ultrasound scan is normal, no follow-up is needed. The general practitioner should be sent a standard letter advising that they have been screened by ultrasound, but still require follow-up until they are observed to be walking with a normal gait.

If any of the above children have minor abnormalities on the ultrasound scan, then they should have a second ultrasound scan 6 weeks later. Children with subluxed or dislocated hips on ultrasound should be seen again in the paediatric orthopaedic clinic.

Any child who has a clinically dislocated or dislocatable hip at birth should have an immediate ultrasound scan and be referred to the next paediatric orthopaedic clinic within a week.

Management of abnormal hips

Apart from cases of irreducible hip dislocation, an infant with a dislocated or dislocatable hip should have a splint applied at about the age of 2 weeks. Further delay may cause poorer results. The Pavlik harness or variants of the von Rosen splint are used (Figure 8.6). They are made of malleable metal that has been padded and then covered with waterproof material. The splint acts equally on both hips, keeping both thighs flexed and at an optimum degree of abduction. Unless substitution by a larger splint is required, the splint must remain in position continuously for at least 2 months if the hip is dislocatable, or for at least 3 months if it is dislocated at rest. Early consultation and follow-up with an orthopaedic surgeon, who will continue long-term care, is essential.

Before the splint is first applied, the parents must be told exactly what this treatment entails. The mother should be encouraged to continue breastfeeding, even though this may prove awkward initially. The infant should be placed naked on the splint, which has been fashioned so that the posterior cross-bar is grooved to protect the skin over the spine. If the hip is dislocated, the dislocation must first be gently reduced and the thigh held in the abducted position while the splint is carefully applied. Potential pressure points may be protected by inserting pieces of cotton wool or similar material. The mother should be told to replace these when they become wet or soiled without disturbing the splint. The infant's clothes should be put over the splint and not under it.

Once the splint is in place, the infant should be washed, weighed and examined without the splint being removed. The splint will

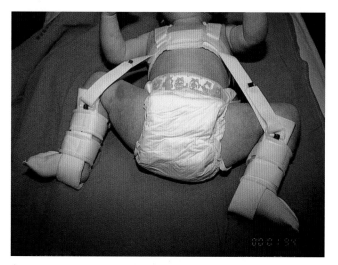

Figure 8.6 Pavlik harness.

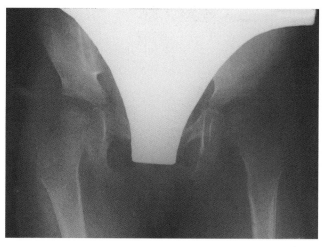

Figure 8.7 Radiograph of normal hips at 18 months.

need scrupulous adjustment at each visit to allow for growth and to ensure that the hip is not being over-abducted. The degree of full abduction in a normal infant diminishes slightly but steadily over the early weeks of life so that the splint should give the comfortable degree of full abduction that is appropriate for the child's age. Failure to adjust progressively for this may cause avascular necrosis of the femoral head. On the other hand, if the degree of thigh abduction is inadequate because the splint is applied too loosely, the hip may remain dislocated.

The splint should be checked daily for several days after application, and thereafter at intervals of not more than 1 or 2 weeks.

Once the splint is finally removed, an anteroposterior radiograph of the hips should be taken with the thighs held parallel, and the infant should be followed up at the ages of 6 and 12 months, at the least.

Late diagnosis

If a dislocated hip is 'missed' in the newborn infant the clinical diagnosis is often difficult until, after some weeks or months, the classic signs of lack of thigh abduction and, in unilateral cases, asymmetry of the lower buttock creases become apparent. Before the age of 4 months an ultrasound scan is the most useful aid to diagnosis. Once ossification occurs in the upper femoral epiphysis

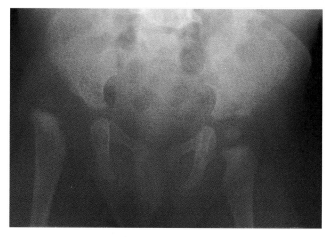

Figure 8.8 Radiograph of dislocated hip at 8 months.

at about the age of 3–4 months, a dislocation can be more clearly shown by radiological examination (Figures 8.7 & 8.8).

Acknowledgement

This chapter was written for the first edition by Dr HVL Finlay and has been revised for each edition.

CHAPTER 9

Infection in the Newborn

OVERVIEW

- Early signs of infection in young infants are often non-specific, particularly if the infant is preterm. Changes in the infant's feeding, behaviour and temperature stability are often more apparent to the parents and experienced nurses.
- Newborn infants are more prone to bacterial infection because of immunological immaturity, and the progression of infection may be very rapid. Newborn infants with apparently minor signs in whom infection cannot be excluded, are therefore often given broad-spectrum systemic antibiotics, at least until the results of the infection screen are known.

Some infections are fulminating and the infant may die within a few hours. More commonly, however, the onset is insidious and the non-specific features may include the refusal of feeds by an infant who has previously fed normally, lethargy, hypotonia, apnoeic attacks or fever (Box 9.1). Fever is arbitrarily defined as a temperature over 37.5°C, but newborn infants with infection often have a normal or even a subnormal temperature.

The most common pathogens in full-term newborn infants are group B streptococci, *Escherichia coli*, *Staphylococcus aureus* and *Pseudomonas aeruginosa*. The pathogens causing infection at a particular site can sometimes be predicted (e.g. *S. aureus* in paronychia) but swabs for bacterial culture should still be taken before giving an antibiotic. Usually an antibiotic needs to be given before the organism has been isolated, but the treatment can be changed later once the sensitivity of the pathogen to antibiotics has been tested in vitro (Figure 9.1). The sensitivity of the pathogens

Box 9.1 **Early signs of neonatal infection**

- Poor feeding or refusal of feeds
- Lethargy
- Hypotonia
- Apnoea
- Fever or hypothermia

ABC of the First Year, Sixth edition. By B. Valman and R. Thomas. © 2009 Blackwell Publishing, ISBN: 978-1-4051-8037-5.

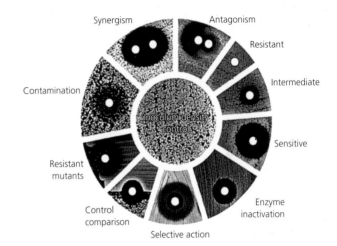

Figure 9.1 Antibiotic disc susceptibility test.

in a particular unit is often known, which may give a guide to effective streatment. If septicaemia is suspected and there is no obvious site of entry of the pathogen, both a penicillin and an aminoglycoside (for example, gentamicin) must be given after a blood culture has been taken.

Intestinal absorption is variable and regurgitation of antibiotics common, so that the intramuscular or intravenous route should always be used initially. Intravenous antibiotics are preferable and should be given slowly by bolus injection rather than by adding them to the bottle of intravenous fluid. Intramuscular injections should be given deeply into the upper lateral aspect of the thigh. Schemes for rotating the sites are essential to prevent local necrosis and to avoid further injections being given into a relatively avascular area.

Group B streptococcal infections

The group B streptococcus is the commonest pathogen that causes severe infection in the first week of life (Box 9.2). It is acquired during birth from the maternal vagina. Although 10–30% of mothers are colonized and about 25% of their infants acquire this organism, fewer than 1 in 1000 infants develop symptoms. About half of those with symptoms die. In the early-onset type of infection, which occurs in the first few days of life, there may be a persistently raised respiratory rate followed by the vague features of septicaemia and later peripheral cyanosis. The chest radiograph may show extensive areas of consolidation in both lungs or it may be normal. The same organism may cause a more insidious septicaemia and meningitis towards the end of the first week.

Parents should be warned that recurrent group B streptococcal infection may occur for up to 3 months after birth and that intravenous antibiotics, given early, are the only effective treatment.

Escherichia coli infections

The use of antibiotics with a wide spectrum of action tends to eliminate all bacteria except *E. coli* and *Pseudomonas*, which flourish in a warm, moist environment. The preterm infant has a greater susceptibility to infection, and nursing in an incubator with increased humidity provides the ideal setting for these infections, especially if broad-spectrum antibiotics are being given. The umbilicus may become infected (Figure 9.2) and this may be followed by septicaemia and later meningitis.

Early symptoms are ill-defined and the nurse may report that the infant appears vaguely unwell. They may have lethargy, anorexia, jaundice and purpura. The early symptoms of meningitis are similar to those of septicaemia, but late features are vomiting, a high-

---

Box 9.2 Group B streptococcal infection

Early onset
Raised respiratory rate
Peripheral cyanosis

Late onset
Insidious septicaemia
Meningitis

---

pitched cry, convulsions, raised anterior fontanelle tension, and rarely neck stiffness.

A urinary tract infection may easily be missed if a specimen of urine is not examined in every infant with fever or who is unwell. Rarely, there are physical signs of an associated congenital abnormality of the urinary tract, such as an enlarged kidney due to hydronephrosis (Figure 9.3) or a persistently palpable bladder and poor urinary stream caused by obstruction from urethral valves in a boy.

Outbreaks of acute gastroenteritis due to rotavirus may occur in newborn nurseries, but these are uncommon if there is attention to scrupulous handwashing by clinical staff and parents.

Staphylococcal infections

Conjunctivitis. Staph. epidermidis is often cultured from eye swabs of infants with conjunctivitis and it is impossible to determine whether this is the primary cause of the conjunctivitis or whether it is secondary to chemical inflammation. Chemicals such as chlorhexidine used in swabbing the mother's perineum may enter the infant's conjunctiva during delivery and cause irritation. Primary infection with *Staph. aureus* may cause severe conjunctivitis. After taking an eye swab from an infant with conjunctivitis, neomycin ophthalmic ointment should be applied to both eyes three times daily for a week.

If mild conjunctivitis persists longer than a week, the possibility of infection with *Chlamydia trachomatis* should be considered. The laboratory may be able to isolate the organism using special techniques. The best treatment consists of a course of tetracycline eye ointment, which should be continued for at least

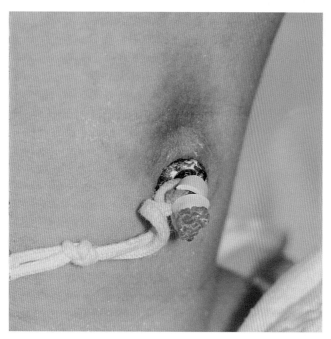

Figure 9.2 Infection (cellulitis) of the umbilicus.

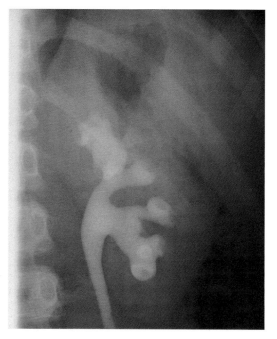

Figure 9.3 Hydronephrosis.

3 weeks and a course of oral erythromycin should also be given for at least 2 weeks in order to prevent recurrence. (See below for gonococcal ophthalmitis.)

Skin sepsis. Clusters of yellow pustules in the axilla or groin that first appear on the fourth day or later are usually due to staphylococci (Figure 9.4). They may resemble the lesions of neonatal erythema, but those lesions appear earlier and resolve within 48 hours. If there is any doubt, the lesions should be treated as staphylococcal pustules.

Bullous impetigo of the newborn is a rare bullous eruption which can be rapidly fatal and very infectious if adequate antibiotics (e.g. intravenous flucloxacillin) are not given (Figure 9.5).

Umbilical infection, shown by a localized red area and a serous exudate, may be due to *Staph. aureus* or a wide variety of other pathogens.

Paronychia is an infection along the side of the fingernail or toenail. It often affects several digits together. The lesion appears trivial, but it may lead to any of the more serious infections due to the staphylococcus. Surgery is not required, but at least a 7-day course of flucloxacillin should be given.

A breast abscess is a red, tender swelling, which may not affect the whole breast; usually there are enlarged lymph nodes in the axilla on the same side (Figure 9.6). Hormonally induced physiological enlargement of the breast (neonatal gynaecomastia) may also be unilateral. Surgical drainage is usually required as well as antibiotics for a breast abscess.

Pneumonia. The signs are the same as those of other types of pneumonia: raised respiratory rate, chest recession and sometimes focal or generalized signs in the lungs. The infant appears extremely ill because of the accompanying septicaemia. A chest radiograph may initially show generalized non-specific changes and later lobar consolidation, occasionally with characteristic pneumatocoeles, which are air-filled spaces. Complications are pneumothorax and empyema, but these are uncommon with early administration of broad-spectrum antibiotics.

In *osteomyelitis,* there are often no specific signs, just an ill infant who will not feed. Reluctance to move a limb and crying when the limb is moved or touched are valuable localizing signs, but swelling at the site of the lesion is a late sign (Figure 9.7). A radioisotope scan may show changes at an early stage of neonatal osteomyelitis and later a radiograph of the limb may show a soft tissue swelling

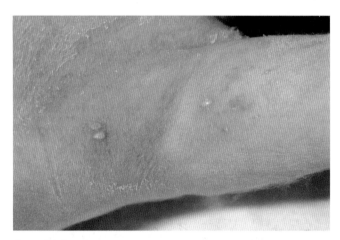

Figure 9.4 Pustules.

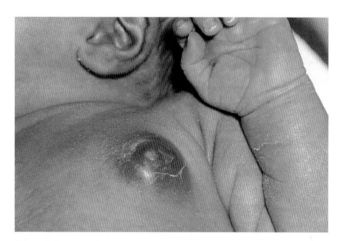

Figure 9.6 Breast abscess.

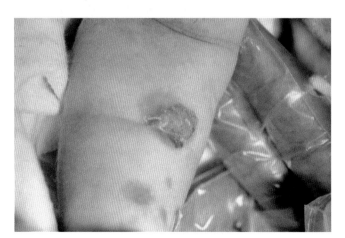

Figure 9.5 Bullous impetigo.

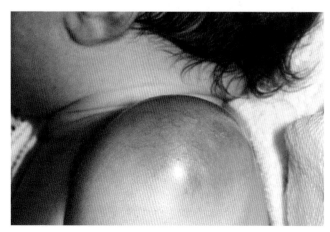

Figure 9.7 Osteomyelitis.

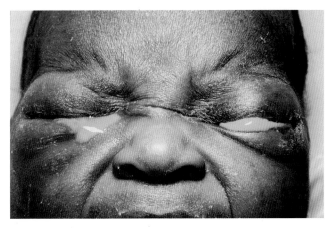

Figure 9.8 Gonococcal ophthalmitis.

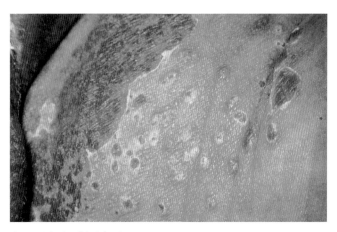

Figure 9.9 *Candida* infection.

or a raised and thickened periosteum. Rarely, osteomyelitis in the newborn is due to organisms other than *Staph. aureus*.

Gonococcal infection

Gonococcal ophthalmitis may be unilateral, usually does not respond completely to local neomycin, and is often present within 24 hours of birth. In cases of severe conjunctivitis, particularly when bilateral and associated with severe oedema, gonococcal infection should be suspected and special arrangements for taking swabs must be made with the laboratory (Figure 9.8). If gonococcal infection is suspected, even if smears do not confirm it, intravenous ceftriaxone or penicillin is given and the diagnosis is reconsidered when the results of the cultures are available. In addition, chloramphenicol eyedrops are given half-hourly for the first 6 hours and then chloramphenicol ointment is applied 2-hourly for 3 days.

If the conjunctivitis does not respond rapidly to treatment, swabs should be taken again for gonococcal infection and for *Chlamydia trachomatis*. The paediatrician should be told as soon as the laboratory confirms the diagnosis in view of the medical and legal implications. Urethral, cervical and rectal swabs should be taken from the mother.

Candida infections (fungal)

Candida infections are encouraged by the widespread or repeated use of broad-spectrum antibiotics. *Candida* infection of the mouth produces white plaques (thrush) and may make the infant reluctant to feed. It also causes a fiery-red scaly eruption of the perineum, usually secondary to ammoniacal dermatitis (Figure 9.9). A swab made damp with sterile sodium chloride solution should be used to obtain a specimen for laboratory confirmation of the cause of the perineal rash. Oral nystatin suspension should be given after feeds for at least a week for the oral lesions. Nystatin ointment should be applied to the perineal rash each time the napkin is changed until the rash has resolved for a week. Miconazole oral gel and miconazole ointment may be used if nystatin suspension is not effective within a few days.

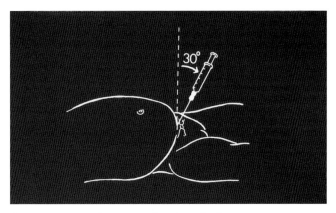

Figure 9.10 Suprapubic puncture for urine collection.

Management and treatment

Careful evaluation of the features noted above may enable a tentative diagnosis to be made and to be confirmed by a single investigation. In many infants, however, there are no specific signs and the following investigations should be carried out.

Urine microscopy and culture. Specimens must be collected carefully and examined promptly to produce reliable results. A fresh midstream clean-catch specimen can often be obtained after gentle suprapubic stimulation, especially in boys. Treatment with systemic antibiotics should not be delayed in an ill infant, so a suprapubic bladder puncture after a feed and with ultrasound guidance is usually the most productive method of obtaining a urine specimen (Figure 9.10). Bacteria cultured from this specimen confirm a urinary tract infection.

Ultrasound renal scan should be performed in all infants with a confirmed urinary tract infection before discharge from the unit to exclude a renal tract obstruction. Arrangements are made for the infant to be reassessed at regular intervals in the outpatient clinic and further investigations may be needed later. Inadequately treated neonatal urinary infections may cause permanent renal scars and later renal failure.

Other investigations that may need to be performed are: (a) culture of gastric aspirate, ear swab and umbilical swab; (b) chest radiograph; (c) blood culture from a peripheral vein, avoiding the femoral vein; and (d) lumbar puncture. After the age of 2 days a blood neutrophil polymorph count higher than 10×10^9/L suggests infection. A very low neutrophil polymorph count also suggests overwhelming infection.

As infants may deteriorate rapidly, treatment is started immediately for the most likely organisms involved if the child is ill. If the infant appears ill, antibiotics suitable for septicaemia should be given intravenously or intramuscularly after all the specimens have been taken. If the diagnosis is uncertain after physical examination, investigation of the urine, chest radiograph and examination of the cerebrospinal fluid (CSF), and the infant appears well, it is better to withhold antibiotics until a paediatrician has been consulted.

Suitable antibiotics are intramuscular or intravenous flucloxacillin for staphylococcal infections, intravenous penicillin for group B streptococcal infections, and intravenous gentamicin for *E. coli* septicaemia (Box 9.3). The combination of intravenous penicillin and gentamicin is appropriate first-line antibiotic treatment for most neonatal infections. Intravenous cefotaxime or ceftriaxone is suitable for *E. coli* meningitis.

To treat urinary tract infection intravenous or intramuscular gentamicin and ampicillin should be given. Once the sensitivities are established, it may be possible to continue treatment with one drug such as trimethoprim. In any case, gentamicin should not be given for longer than a week, as eighth nerve damage may occur. Every infant who has had a confirmed urinary tract infection should have a repeat examination of the urine for the presence of infection every 3 months for 2 years.

Gentamicin is an effective antibiotic which can be given as a once-daily dose, but it can cause deafness if blood levels are excessively high and levels must be monitored. The serum concentrations of gentamicin should be between 5 and 10 mg/L 1 hour after the previous dose. The trough blood level, taken just before the next dose is due, should be less than 2 mg/L.

Paediatric HIV

Perinatal transmission of HIV from an infected mother to her infant can now be reduced to below 1% by preventive measures taken during pregnancy and the perinatal period. It is recommended that all mothers are encouraged to have an HIV screening test as part of their routine antenatal screening. It is now known that infants are most at risk of becoming infected with HIV during vaginal delivery, when they swallow maternal secretions containing the virus and later during breastfeeding. The administration of highly active anti-retroviral therapy (HAART) to the mother during pregnancy is not harmful to the fetus and, together with elective caesarean section, avoidance of breastfeeding, and the administration of AZT (zidovudine) to the infant, has been shown to reduce the rate of vertical transmission from 15–30% to <1% in countries where these measures are safe and affordable. The risk of transmission is related to maternal viral load in the third trimester and if this is undetectable in mothers who are on HAART, caesarean section may not confer any additional benefit.

Although breastfeeding doubles the rate of vertical transmission, in developing countries it may still be the preferred method of infant feeding because of the greater health risks associated with formula feeding.

All infants born to HIV-positive mothers will also test HIV antibody positive for at least the first 12–18 months of life, even those who are uninfected, because of the passage of maternal antibodies (IgG) across the placenta to the baby. Uninfected infants can usually be identified by showing absence of the virus on at least 2–3 tests by polymerase chain reaction (PCR) in the first 4 months of life. Until the results of the PCR tests are known, infants born to mothers who have a detectable viral load prior to delivery will be given oral co-trimoxazole (daily or at least three times a week) from 1 month of age, in order to prevent infection with *Pneumocystis carinii*, which can cause a severe life-threatening pneumonia (PCP) in infected infants. Routine immunization with the triple, Hib and meningococcal vaccines should be given at the usual age. Some paediatricians recommend intramuscular polio instead of oral polio vaccine for the infant, in order to avoid the small risk of immunocompromised adults in the family developing poliomyelitis. BCG vaccination is usually delayed until the infant is confirmed to be uninfected with HIV.

Infants infected with HIV may remain asymptomatic for 10–12 years after birth but around 20% will develop serious problems in the first year of life. Recurrent thrush, skin rashes, lymphadenopathy (Figure 9.11), hepatosplenomegaly, failure to thrive, developmental delay and severe respiratory tract infections are common symptoms in HIV-positive infants (Box 9.4). HAART is only necessary when the infant is shown to have a high viral load and a low number of CD4 lymphocytes. The survival of infected children has been greatly improved by early diagnosis and treatment, but there is no definitive cure for HIV-infected individuals as yet.

Families with HIV, even those where the children are not infected, benefit from support and help from sympathetic, well-informed healthcare professionals.

Common napkin rashes

Napkin rashes are usually due to ammoniacal dermatitis, seborrhoeic dermatitis or perianal excoriation.

Ammoniacal dermatitis is caused by ammonia produced by faecal bacterial enzymes acting on urea in the urine. Erythema,

---

Box 9.3 **Antibiotics for specific infections**

- Staphylococcus   Flucloxacillin
- Streptococcus   Benzylpenicillin (i.v.)
- *E. coli*
  - Septicaemia   Gentamicin
  - Meningitis   Cefotaxime or ceftriaxone

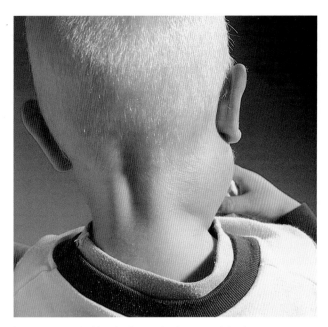

Figure 9.11 Cervical lymphadenopathy due to HIV infection.

Box 9.4 **Clinical features of HIV**

- Recurrent *Candida* infection
- Generalized lymphadenopathy
- Parotitis
- Failure to thrive
- Pneumocystis pneumonia
- Developmental delay

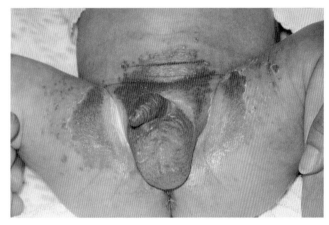

Figure 9.12 Ammoniacal dermatitis.

papules, scaling and erosions appear in areas that have been in contact with napkins soaked with urine (Figure 9.12). The depths of the skin folds are spared, and the prepuce and scrotum are especially vulnerable. The principle of treatment is to keep urine and faeces away from the skin. Initial treatment includes changing napkins frequently or leaving the child without a napkin whenever feasible. A protective barrier cream is applied to the affected area

every time the napkin is changed; in resistant cases a silicone cream is used. Some authorities consider that the formation of ammonia does not play a major part in this condition and they prefer the term 'irritant napkin dermatitis'.

If the rash does not improve within 10 days, *Candida* infection of the lesions should be considered. This rash has a fiery red appearance with a scaly edge, often with a few early papules separated from the main eruption. Nystatin cream should be applied to the rash each time the napkin is changed for at least a week. The infant's mouth should be examined to determine whether white plaques of *Candida* are present and an oral suspension of nystatin is needed. Alternatively, miconazole oral gel may be used. In breastfed infants the mother's nipples should be examined, as a scaling dermatitis of the nipples can be due to *Candida* and may reinfect the infant.

Any infant with a rash in the napkin area should be undressed completely to ensure that he or she does not have a rash elsewhere. In seborrhoeic dermatitis the erythema and scaling may also affect the axillae, neck, area behind the ears, scalp, forehead and eyelids (Figure 9.13). The scalp may be covered with adherent hard crusted plaques (cradle cap). Secondary infection by staphylococci, streptococci or *Candida* is common. The condition always begins before

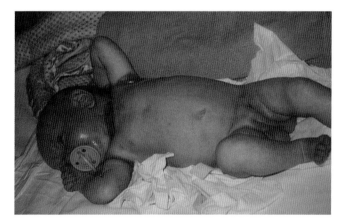

Figure 9.13 Seborrhoeic dermatitis.

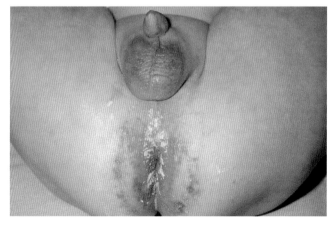

Figure 9.14 Perianal excoriation.

the age of 3 months and clears completely without treatment by 9 months. In contrast to the infant with ammoniacal dermatitis who has discomfort in association with the rash, the infant with seborrhoeic dermatitis is oblivious of the rash. The cause is unknown and there is usually no family history of dermatitis. Treatment with 1% hydrocortisone ointment is rapidly effective and the lesions usually clear completely within a few weeks. In severe cases nystatin or an antibacterial agent may be added to the cream. Cradle cap can be removed by shampoo containing 0.5% salicylic acid.

If the rash affects mainly the perianal area, it is probably due to persistently loose stools. Perianal excoriation is commonly found in infants with gastroenteritis and resolves when the diarrhoea stops (Figure 9.14). Zinc cream or exposure may hasten the resolution of the lesions, but changes in the stool pH and consistency are the most important factors.

Further reading

Rennie JM. (2005) *Robertson's Textbook of Neonatology,* 4th edn. Churchill Livingstone, Edinburgh.

CHAPTER 10

Jaundice in the Newborn

OVERVIEW

- Mild jaundice is common after the first 48 hours of age but most infants do not require any special investigation or treatment

- Jaundice that starts early, particularly within the first 24 hours of life, is most likely to be due to haemolytic disease or infection. Rhesus haemolytic disease is now very uncommon as mothers who are rhesus negative are routinely given anti-D at 28 and 34 weeks gestation

- Prolonged jaundice beyond 14 days of age in a full-term infant requires investigation to exclude conditions that may cause serious problems if they are not diagnosed and treated early (e.g. hypothyroidism, galactosaemia, biliary atresia). Some infants who are exclusively breastfed have prolonged jaundice, but this does not require cessation of breastfeeding

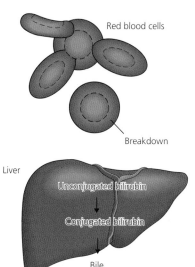

Figure 10.1 Formation and excretion of bilirubin.

Jaundice is a yellow colour of the skin caused by a high concentration of bilirubin (Figure 10.1). Very severe jaundice may damage the cells of the basal ganglia and brainstem. This damage is produced by the fat-soluble unconjugated bilirubin. If jaundice is severe, high bilirubin levels may result in deafness, cerebral palsy or death.

Neonatal jaundice is due to an increased bilirubin load with a transient inefficiency of hepatic excretion resulting from decreased activity of glucuronyl transferase in the liver. There are additional factors. Some of the conjugated bilirubin excreted in the bile is normally deconjugated in the small intestine and reabsorption is enhanced by the slower gut transit in the newborn who takes small volumes of milk. Bilirubin is absorbed from meconium and there is no intestinal flora to degrade bilirubin to urobilinogen.

Jaundice in the skin is visible to the naked eye in white Caucasian infants at a serum bilirubin level of about 80 μmol/L. In black infants the sclerae should be examined as jaundice is more difficult to recognise. Jaundice first appears in the face and spreads to the periphery of the limbs. The level is more than 270 μmol/L if the hands or feet are jaundiced (Figure 10.2).

Common causes of jaundice in the newborn (Box 10.1)

Common causes of jaundice include hepatic immaturity, red cell incompatibility, infection and breastfeeding (Figure 10.3).

Jaundice due to hepatic immaturity, or 'physiological' jaundice, is common in both preterm and full-term babies. A temporary deficiency of glucuronyl transferase enzymes reduces the rate of conjugation of bilirubin, with a consequent retention of unconjugated bilirubin. In full-term infants physiological jaundice appears after the first 24 hours of life and reaches a peak on the fourth or fifth day. In preterm infants it usually begins 48 hours after birth and may last up to 2 weeks.

In babies with red cell incompatibility, jaundice appears within 24 hours of birth. The main causes are (a) incompatible rhesus grouping and (b) incompatible ABO grouping; the mother's blood is usually group O and the infant's group A or, less commonly, group B.

The common infective causes of jaundice are septicaemia and urinary tract infection. Septicaemia is especially likely to be present if the jaundice appears after the fourth day of life, but it is a possibility in any infant who seems ill. In urinary tract infections, the jaundice is of hepatic origin.

ABC of the First Year, Sixth edition. By B. Valman and R. Thomas. © 2009 Blackwell Publishing, ISBN: 978-1-4051-8037-5.

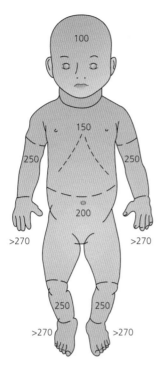

Figure 10.2 Spread of jaundice in the skin.

Box 10.1 **Causes of jaundice**

Cause	Onset
Red cell incompatibility	Within 24 hours of birth
Physiological jaundice	After 24 hours
Septicaemia	At any age but usually after fourth day

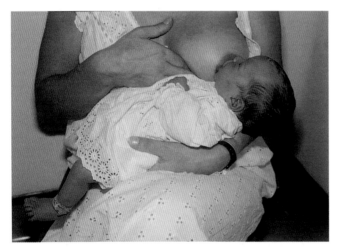

Figure 10.3 Breastfeeding.

In about 2.5% of infants who are breastfed the serum bilirubin rises to levels of between 260 and 360 µmol/L in the second or third week of life. These infants have no symptoms. If breastfeeding continues, the level remains constant for 3 or 4 weeks and falls to

Box 10.2 **Rare causes of jaundice**

- Hypothyroidism
- Galactosaemia
- Viral hepatitis
- Atresia of bile ducts
- Glucose-6-phosphate dehydrogenase deficiency

normal levels by 4–16 weeks. An abnormal progesterone has been shown in the milk of some mothers.

Rare causes of jaundice in the newborn

Rare causes of jaundice include hypothyroidism, galactosaemia, viral hepatitis and atresia of the bile ducts (Box 10.2). These cause prolonged jaundice lasting more than 10 days. Glucose-6-phosphate dehydrogenase deficiency is another cause of prolonged jaundice, but it can also produce a clinical picture similar to blood group incompatibility.

In hypothyroidism, physiological jaundice is prolonged, the plasma thyroxine (T4) concentration is reduced, and the thyroid-stimulating hormone (TSH) concentration is increased.

In infants with viral hepatitis, which is usually due to intra-uterine infection, the stools are pale, the urine dark owing to bile, and there is a high level of conjugated bilirubin in the plasma.

It is difficult to differentiate between hepatitis and atresia of the bile ducts clinically, and they may represent the two ends of a spectrum of disease. If jaundice persists more than 10 days, the advice of a paediatrician should be sought.

In galactosaemia the urine gives a positive result on testing for reducing substances, but the test for glucose may be negative. The infant needs to be referred to a paediatrician immediately for special investigations.

Glucose-6-phosphate dehydrogenase deficiency occurs in infants of Mediterranean, African, or Chinese origin. This hereditary red cell enzyme defect is found in male infants with haemolytic episodes that often occur without the usual precipitating factors of drugs or infection. The enzyme is necessary for maintaining the stability of the red cell membrane.

Management of jaundice starting in the first 24 hours

If jaundice appears within 24 hours of birth, it must be considered to be due to blood group incompatibility until proved otherwise. There is a high risk of cerebral palsy unless the jaundice is managed appropriately. Most rhesus haemolytic disease problems should be anticipated before the neonatal period by antenatal maternal screening. Urgent exchange transfusion may be indicated in infants severely affected by haemolytic disease of the newborn, and it is advisable for the infant to be admitted to hospital immediately for investigation and management. If the mother is rhesus negative, she will have been given antenatal intramuscular anti-D to reduce the risk of haemolytic disease in the rhesus-positive infant.

A positive Coombs test in a rhesus-positive infant of a rhesus-negative mother who has received anti-D within 4–6 weeks of delivery cannot be used to confirm the diagnosis of rhesus incompatibility, which must be made on the basis of rate of rise of plasma bilirubin and falling haemoglobin in the infant. The plasma bilirubin concentration should be measured every 4–8 hours and the results plotted on a special chart (see page 53). Once the second estimation has been performed the maximum concentration can be predicted, as the rate of increase is linear. When the serial concentrations fall below the printed line, the infant is unlikely to need any treatment.

Management of jaundice starting after the first 24 hours (Box 10.3)

The possibility of septicaemia or urinary tract infection should be considered in any ill baby who develops jaundice after the first 24 hours of life. If there is any doubt about when the jaundice first appeared, the possibility of blood group incompatibility should be investigated.

When a doctor or midwife sees the infant on the postnatal ward or at home, a guide to the plasma bilirubin concentration can be provided by the hand-held dermal icterometer which can be used for infants of any gestation and any skin colour or racial origin. A disposable sensor is pressed gently on the infant's forehead and gives the combined total of conjugated and unconjugated bilirubin in the blood flowing to the skin (Figure 10.4). A laboratory plasma bilirubin should always be checked if the infant is already having phototherapy or if the hand-held icterometer shows a level over 200 mmol/L (Figure 10.4).

In full-term infants if the dermal icterometer suggests that the plasma bilirubin concentration is about 250 µmol/L or the result lies above the line on the chart the infant should be transferred to hospital immediately. If the plasma bilirubin level is very high, urgent exchange transfusion or phototherapy may be needed (Figure 10.5).

In neonatal units there is usually a ward bilirubinometer that measures plasma bilirubin concentrations within a few minutes, using a small specimen of blood obtained by heel prick. If two estimations fall below the line on the chart, treatment will probably not be needed. Those with values above the line may need exposure to ultraviolet light under a phototherapy unit (Figure 10.6). Phototherapy produces geometric stereoisomers of bilirubin, which

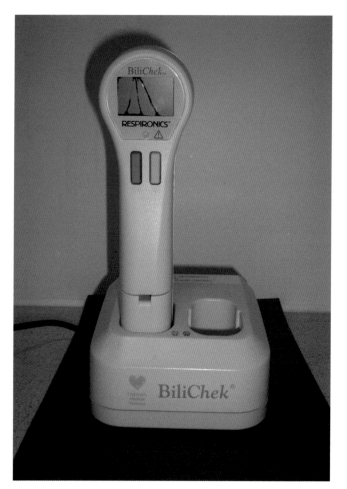

Figure 10.4 Dermal icterometer.

have no known long-term deleterious effect on the infant, but the parents should have the procedure explained first. The infant's eyes are shielded with eye pads. Although phototherapy units have a shield to reduce transfer of heat from the lamp to the infant, monitoring of the temperature of the infant is essential. Extra fluids may be needed to compensate for the additional evaporative loss and this can be given as additional breast milk (or formula to bottle-fed babies). Milk stimulates gut motility and improves the excretion of bilirubin and the associated compounds.

The indications for phototherapy are controversial, but many units give phototherapy if the plasma bilirubin level is above the line on the chart. Despite phototherapy, an exchange transfusion may still be needed, but the critical level varies with the unit, the gestational age and the general condition of the infant. Exchange transfusion should be considered if the plasma bilirubin level exceeds 450 µmol/L in a full-term infant and 300 µmol/L in a preterm infant. Some units start treatment at lower levels of bilirubin in sick infants.

Prolonged jaundice

If jaundice persists longer than 14 days in a full-term infant, blood should be taken for plasma thyroxine and TSH estimations and

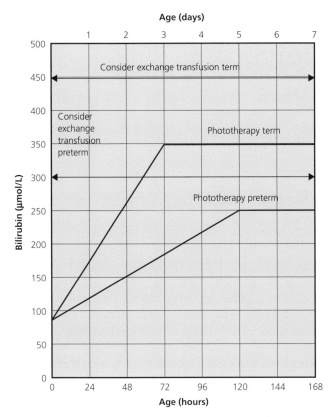

Figure 10.5 Indications for phototherapy and exchange transfusion.

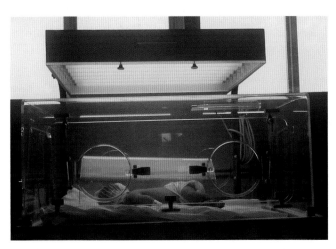

Figure 10.6 Phototherapy.

Box 10.4 **Prolonged jaundice >14 days**

- Serum bilirubin – conjugated and unconjugated
- Full blood count
- Thyroid function tests
- Liver enzymes
- Glucose-6-phosphate dehydrogenase
- Urine culture
- Urine for reducing substances (for galactosaemia)
- Urine for presence of bilirubin which reflects a high conjugated bilirubin (on a Labstix)

a specimen of urine collected to test for reducing substances and glucose (Box 10.4). The urine should be examined in the laboratory for the presence of infection. If the parents are of Mediterranean, African or Chinese origin, the screening test for red cell glucose-6-phosphate dehydrogenase should also be performed.

Pale stools and a plasma conjugated bilirubin level greater than 30 μmol/L suggest the possibility of hepatitis or atresia of the bile ducts, and the advice of a paediatrician is needed.

If there is a suspicion that the jaundice is related to breastfeeding, the other conditions causing jaundice should be excluded and the mother advised to continue breastfeeding. If the plasma bilirubin concentration is rising rapidly and breastfeeding is stopped for 48 hours, the infant's plasma bilirubin concentration will fall abruptly and will not usually rise on return to breastfeeding. Although the mother can continue lactation by expressing her milk during this diagnostic test, there is a risk that breastfeeding will not be resumed, so it is rarely recommended.

Further reading

Rennie JM. (2005) *Robertson's Textbook of Neonatology,* 4th edn. Churchill Livingstone, Edinburgh.

Convulsions in the Newborn

Although the involuntary movements of a convulsion in the newborn are usually generalized, they may affect only one limb, the face or the tongue. The distinctive feature is repetitive jerky movements, which may be accompanied by loss of consciousness, apnoea or rigidity (Figure 11.1). Often the convulsion has stopped by the time the baby is seen by a doctor. A brisk Moro reflex or jerky normal movements in a baby may be misinterpreted as a convulsion by an inexperienced observer. Myoclonic jerks occur in healthy infants, usually in association with sleep, and can be differentiated from convulsions by the abolition of the abnormal movements when the infant is given something to suck or when the jerking limb is held firmly by the examiner. If the convulsion is not witnessed, apnoea or cyanosis may indicate that it has occurred, and if there is any doubt it is safer to investigate the baby on the assumption that there has been a convulsion.

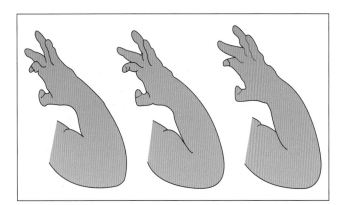

Figure 11.1 Repetitive similar movements indicate a convulsion.

ABC of the First Year, Sixth edition. By B. Valman and R. Thomas. © 2009 Blackwell Publishing, ISBN: 978-1-4051-8037-5.

Management

A baby not already in hospital should be admitted. The infant is placed on his or her side and the airway cleared by suction of the pharynx under direct vision. The baby should be nursed in an incubator to improve observation. Oxygen is given in high concentration with a funnel or head box until the convulsion has stopped.

After hypoglycaemia has been excluded by a blood glucose estimation, an anticonvulsant should be given if the convulsion is continuing or recurs while waiting for the results of other investigations. The order of carrying out the various procedures is important. Hypoglycaemia and hypocalcaemia should each be sought for and excluded in that order before the next test (Box 11.1). Hypoglycaemia is the more dangerous condition. If the plasma glucose and calcium concentrations are normal, a paediatrician should decide whether a lumbar puncture is indicated (Box 11.2).

Hypoglycaemia

A specimen of blood should be taken immediately from a heel prick for glucose measurement in a ward or cot-side glucometer (Figure 11.2). If the value is less than 3.0 mmol/L, hypoglycaemia may be present. A further blood sample should be taken and part

Box 11.1 Common causes of neonatal convulsions

- Hypoglycaemia
- Hypocalcaemia
- Cerebral oedema
- Hypoxic ischaemic encephalopathy

Box 11.2 Less common causes of neonatal convulsions

- Hypomagnesaemia
- Pyridoxine deficiency
- Intracerebral haemorrhage
- Neonatal stroke
- Meningitis
- Encephalitis
- Developmental disorders of the brain
- Epilepsy

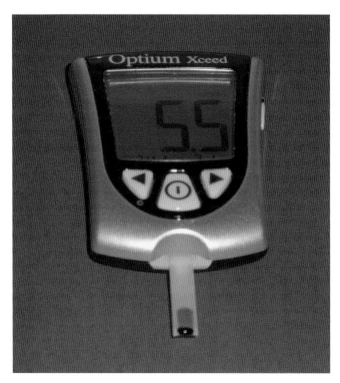

Figure 11.2 Glucometer.

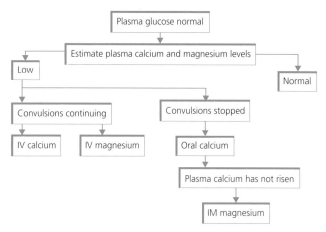

Figure 11.3 Biochemical investigation of a convulsion.

of it used to repeat the glucometer test and the remainder taken into a fluoride tube for the laboratory to check the blood glucose concentration. Hypoglycaemia is defined as a laboratory-estimated blood glucose level of less than 2.6 mmol/L. If the second glucometer value is low, 5 mL of 10% glucose solution per kg body weight should immediately be given intravenously slowly into a limb vein. A continuous intravenous infusion of 10% glucose solution is then set up, initially at a rate of 60 mL/kg a day.

Hypoglycaemia accompanied by convulsions is treated with intravenous glucose to restore normoglycaemia, and when the convulsions have ceased, frequent or continuous intragastric milk should be given.

The amount of intravenous glucose should be reduced gradually over at least 24 hours. During this period, 3-hourly glucometer tests are carried out, supplemented by regular laboratory blood glucose measurements. If an intravenous infusion of glucose is stopped suddenly by accident, severe reactive hypoglycaemia may follow and cause severe convulsions.

Healthy term infants, particularly those who are breastfed, may have asymptomatic hypoglycaemia in the first few days after birth. Random or routine blood glucose screening in low-risk, asymptomatic healthy infants is of no benefit and may lead to unnecessary treatment.

Hypocalcaemia

If the glucometer test result is normal, blood should be taken for emergency plasma calcium estimation (Figure 11.3). If convulsions are still occurring or recur after hypoglycaemia has been excluded by the glucometer, intramuscular paraldehyde should be given while the results of detailed tests are awaited. If the plasma calcium

concentration is lower than 1.8 mmol/L (7 mg/100 mL) treatment depends on whether the convulsions are still occurring or recurring. If the convulsions have stopped, 1–2 mL of 10% calcium gluconate is added to each feed. The calcium gluconate should be added to the feed and not given directly to the infant. The total dose of calcium gluconate in 24 hours should not exceed 12 mL of the 10% solution in the full-term infant.

If the convulsions continue and the plasma calcium concentration is low, 10% calcium gluconate should be diluted to 2.5% with 5% glucose solution in a syringe and given slowly intravenously into a limb or umbilical vein until the convulsions cease or until a maximum of 4 mL/kg body weight of the 2.5% diluted solution has been given. The heart rate is monitored with a cardiac monitor or stethoscope during the procedure and the injection stopped if bradycardia occurs. Calcium gluconate should be added to the feeds until the plasma calcium concentration rises to normal. Calcium gluconate must never be given intramuscularly or allowed to escape out of a vein as severe tissue necrosis may occur.

Intravenous calcium may not control hypocalcaemic convulsions immediately. Some authorities have found that hypocalcaemic convulsions are treated effectively by intramuscular magnesium sulphate (0.2 mL/kg of a 10% solution/dose).

Hypomagnesaemia

Hypocalcaemia may be associated with low plasma magnesium concentrations. If there are recurrent fits or the plasma calcium concentration does not rise despite supplementary calcium gluconate, the plasma magnesium concentration should be estimated. If this is less than 0.6 mmol/L (1.5 mg/100 mL), intramuscular or intravenous magnesium sulphate is given. The dose is 0.2 mL/kg of a 10% solution given intramuscularly every 6 hours; if the plasma level is normal no further treatment is needed. The plasma estimation must be repeated after 2 days. The main toxic effect is hypotonia, which can be reversed by intravenous calcium gluconate if the features are severe.

Prognosis

Hypoglycaemia and hypocalcaemia may be found together, especially in infants of diabetic mothers, but hypoglycaemia is the more

Box 11.3 **Prognosis**

- Symptomatic hypoglycaemia: cautious prognosis
- Symptomatic hypocalcaemia: good prognosis

dangerous (Box 11.3). Symptomatic hypoglycaemia may be followed by mental impairment, but asymptomatic hypocalcaemia or hypomagnesaemia has an excellent prognosis. Enamel hypoplasia, which predisposes to dental caries, is a rare, late complication of hypocalcaemia. Intravenous glucose is not hazardous provided that the correct dose is given, but rapid infusion of intravenous calcium salts may lead to cardiac arrest.

Cerebral lesions

After hypoglycaemia and hypocalcaemia have been excluded, meningitis, intracranial haemorrhage and cerebral oedema due to perinatal hypoxia or ischaemia should be considered. Lethargy, hypotonia and raised tension of the anterior fontanelle are suggestive of a cerebral cause, but meningitis may be present with no specific symptoms or signs. Lumbar puncture is indicated if there is a possibility of meningitis. Ultrasound examination is reliable in excluding an intraventricular or large intracerebral haemorrhage, but may not detect a small subarachnoid or subdural haemorrhage.

If the first convulsion is prolonged or the convulsion recurs, intravenous phenobarbitone should be given. The initial dose of phenobarbitone is 15 mg/kg given intravenously over half an hour. The maintenance dose is started 24 hours later and is usually required for only 2 or 3 days.

Further reading

Rennie JM. (2005) *Robertson's Textbook of Neonatology*, 4th edn. Churchill Livingstone, Edinburgh.

CHAPTER 12

Vomiting

OVERVIEW

- Vomiting should be distinguished from regurgitation
- The material vomited – frothy mucoid, bile-stained or bloodstained – may indicate specific diagnoses
- Vomiting after the first week is often due to a feeding problem or gastro-oesophageal reflux but infections and pyloric stenosis should be considered

Vomiting in the newborn: types of vomit

Vomiting is the forceful expulsion of gastric contents through the mouth. Mothers often confuse vomiting with mild regurgitation, which is the effortless bringing up of small amounts of milk during and between feeds, usually accompanied by air, and is of no importance. If the milk dribbles down the chest it is likely to be regurgitation. Recurrent vomiting may be a sign of lethal disease, but a careful history and examination enable a diagnosis to be made with the minimum of special investigations.

Frothy mucoid vomit

Oesophageal atresia with tracheo-oesophageal fistula may present with vomiting, coughing and cyanosis when the infant begins the first feed. Many of these infants drool frothy material continuously rather than vomit. Vomiting of frothy mucoid material may be the only definite observation, but the condition should be suspected in any baby who has any symptoms during the first feed. As the fluid expelled is not gastric contents, vomiting is not an accurate description but this is the term often used.

Bile-stained vomit

The vomit in infants with intestinal obstruction is usually yellow due to bile staining, but occasionally it consists only of milk. The cause may be atresia, stenosis or volvulus of the small gut, necrotizing enterocolitis, or congenital intestinal aganglionosis (Hirschsprung's disease) of the large gut (Figure 12.1). Abdominal distension is usually present and there may be visible

ABC of the First Year, Sixth edition. By B. Valman and R. Thomas. © 2009 Blackwell Publishing, ISBN: 978-1-4051-8037-5.

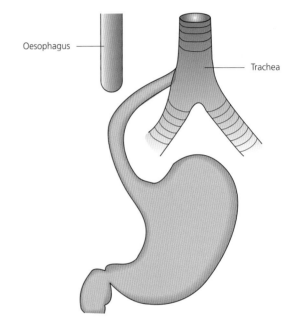

Oesophagus

Trachea

Figure 12.1 Oesophageal atresia with tracheo-oesophageal fistula.

peristalsis. A plain radiograph should be taken in the erect position immediately (Figure 12.2). An alternative is a radiograph in the supine position and, in addition a lateral view with the baby lying on his or her back and a horizontal X-ray beam. They often show fluid levels, dilated loops of gut proximal to the obstruction, and the absence of gas shadows distally. Ideally, every infant who vomits bile should be seen by a surgeon within an hour.

Bloodstained vomit

Bloodstained vomit may be caused by trauma from a feeding tube, swallowed maternal blood or, most seriously, haemorrhagic disease of the newborn. Trauma caused by a feeding tube may produce a few specks of blood in the vomit. Maternal blood may be swallowed before delivery after premature separation of the placenta or after delivery as the result of bleeding from a cracked nipple. Maternal haemoglobin in the vomit can be recognized in the laboratory.

Haemorrhagic disease of the newborn begins between the second and fourth days of life in the early type or in the third or fourth week in the late type. The first symptom may be haematemesis or melaena and the bleeding can be profuse. An immediate

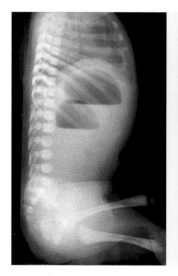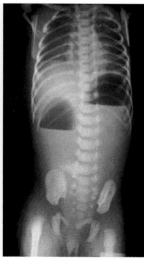

Figure 12.2 Erect lateral (left) and anteroposterior (right) radiographs to show fluid levels.

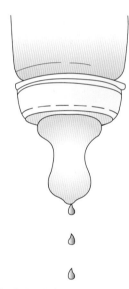

Figure 12.3 Drops of milk should follow quickly and there should not be a continuous stream.

dose of 1 mg vitamin K_1 should be given intramuscularly and a transfusion of fresh blood given urgently if bleeding has been severe or persists after vitamin K treatment.

Milk

Vomiting of milk may be caused by infections, feeding problems, necrotizing enterocolitis, intracranial haemorrhage or drugs. Gastroenteritis, urinary tract infection, septicaemia and meningitis may all be associated with vomiting. A ravenous infant may swallow excessive air at the beginning of the feed and, if not properly 'winded', may later regurgitate milk with air. Larger feeds, more frequent feeds, or a larger hole in the teat is needed (Figure 12.3).

Necrotizing enterocolitis occurs in epidemics in neonatal baby units. Lethargy and refusal of feeds are followed by vomiting and abdominal distension. In the majority of the infants

---

Box 12.1 **Vomiting after the first week**

- Feeding problems
- Infections:
    Urinary tract infection
    Septicaemia
    Meningitis

---

there is blood in the stool. Predisposing factors are prematurity, perinatal hypoxia, hypotension, umbilical vessel catheterization and prolonged rupture of the membranes. Embolism or thrombosis of mesenteric vessels is followed by ischaemic changes, which vary from mucosal ulceration to complete necrosis of the gut wall. Bacteria invade the necrotic tissue and healing is followed by scarring and sometimes a stricture. Despite optimal treatment there is a 25% mortality rate and early advice from a paediatric surgeon is advisable.

Raised intracranial pressure due to intracranial haemorrhage may cause vomiting of milk, as may several drugs.

Vomiting from the first week to the first year: causes

As in the newborn, vomiting in infants older than 1 week may be a symptom of a feeding problem or an infection such as urinary tract infection, otitis media, gastroenteritis, septicaemia or meningitis (Box 12.1; see also page 105).

If no cause of the vomiting is found and the symptoms are mild, urine should be collected for microscopy and culture and should be examined for protein, bile and reducing substances.

Pyloric stenosis

Pyloric stenosis must be considered in every infant less than 3 months of age who vomits. Rarely the vomiting may occur in the first week of life, but it usually begins in the second or third week, though there may be a delay before the infant is seen by a doctor. Usually the vomit is produced forcefully and reaches some distance from the infant. The infant often accepts another feed immediately after vomiting. Stools are infrequent. If the symptoms have been present for more than a few days, there will be a loss of weight due to dehydration and loss of subcutaneous fat. Scanty urine is associated with dehydration.

The essential diagnostic sign is the presence of a pyloric mass palpated during a test feed. Constant practice is needed to appreciate a pyloric mass. Even if no pyloric mass is felt during the first test feed, if the diagnosis of pyloric stenosis is probable the infant should be admitted for rehydration and the examination repeated. Preliminary aspiration and measurement of gastric contents is helpful, particularly if no feed has been given during the preceding 4 hours. Metabolic alkalosis strongly suggests the diagnosis.

In a small proportion of infants the diagnosis of pyloric stenosis is suspected clinically but no pyloric mass is palpable during a test feed. The diagnosis may be confirmed, preferably by an ultrasound study. A barium study is needed rarely.

Intestinal obstruction

Infants who vomit greenish yellow bile are likely to have intestinal obstruction. They should be admitted immediately and seen by a surgeon within an hour. Abdominal distension is often present and peristalsis may be visible. Duodenal stenosis usually presents during the first few days of life but malrotation of the gut with associated volvulus may produce symptoms at any time during childhood.

An inguinal hernia is more likely to incarcerate in the early months of life than later (Figure 12.4). Incarceration should be suspected if the hernia is tender or is not reduced easily. The infant should be seen by a surgeon immediately. The risk of obstruction is always present and early surgical treatment is advisable in every baby with an inguinal hernia. The baby must remain in the ward until the operation is performed.

An intussusception is a partial or complete intestinal obstruction due to invagination of a portion of the gut into a more distal portion (Figure 12.5). It may occur at any age, although the maximum incidence is at 3–11 months. An intussusception may be easily diagnosed in a child who has all the typical features, but these children are not common. The distinctive feature is the

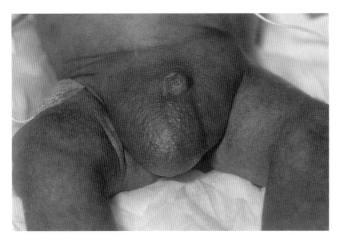

Figure 12.4 Bilateral inguinal hernias.

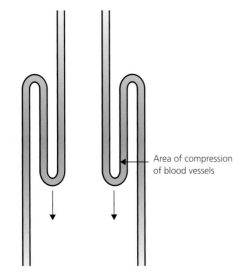

Area of compression
of blood vessels

Figure 12.5 Intussusception.

periodicity of the attacks, which may consist of severe screaming, drawing up of the legs and severe pallor. Some episodes consist of pallor alone. The attack lasts a few minutes and may recur about 20 minutes later, though attacks may be more frequent. There may be vomiting and one or two loose stools may be passed initially, suggesting acute gastroenteritis. Bloodstained mucus may be passed rectally or shown by rectal examination, but some patients pass no blood rectally. Between attacks the infant appears normal and may have no abnormal signs apart from a palpable mass.

It is difficult to examine the abdomen during an attack because the child cries continuously, but between attacks a mass, most commonly over the right upper quadrant, can be felt in 70% of children.

If surgical shock is present, then rapid resuscitation should be carried out and intravenous fluids, including blood, given. Plain radiograph of the abdomen may show evidence of intestinal obstruction or a density in the area of the lesion. Ultrasound may show a doughnut configuration with hypoechogenic rims and a dense central echogenic core. An urgent surgical opinion should be obtained. If the symptoms have been present for less than 48 hours and there are no signs of intestinal perforation, an air or barium enema should be given urgently while the surgeon remains nearby. In over 75% of cases it is possible to reduce the intussusception by the enema. If the intussusception is not reduced, then immediate laparotomy is needed to reduce the lesion manually or to perform an intestinal resection. In about 6% of cases there is a persisting mechanical cause of the intussusception and this will not be detected by the enema.

Gastro-oesophageal reflux

Vomiting due to gastro-oesophageal reflux starts during the first week of life and the vomitus may be bloodstained. Aspiration into the lungs may cause recurrent bronchospasm and severe vomiting may cause failure to thrive, dysphagia, or stricture formation (Box 12.2). During the first year the lower oesophageal sphincter pressure increases and oesophageal mobility becomes more organized. These factors reduce the regurgitation of gastric contents into the oesophagus when the intra-abdominal pressure rises, for example during crying.

The diagnosis can be confirmed by 24-hour pH monitoring of the lower oesophagus. A probe the size of a nasogastric tube is placed just above the gastro-oesophageal sphincter. The pH recording is analysed by computer. Barium swallow examination is often negative despite typical symptoms.

Vomiting usually resolves by the age of 1 year without specific treatment. If symptoms are severe, the feeds can be thickened with ground rice or carob seed powder and infants may be put down

Box 12.2 **Features of gastro-oesophageal reflux**

- Vomiting
- Aspiration
- Failure to thrive
- Dysphagia
- Stenosis (rare)

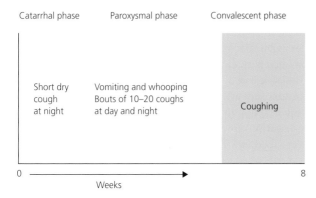

Catarrhal phase   Paroxysmal phase   Convalescent phase

Short dry cough at night

Vomiting and whooping Bouts of 10–20 coughs at day and night

Coughing

0 ——————————————→ 8

Weeks

Figure 12.6 Phases of whooping cough.

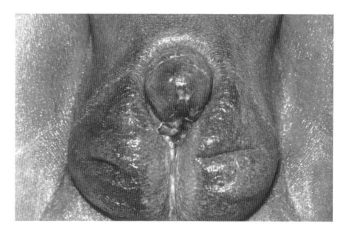

Figure 12.7 Adrenogenital syndrome.

to sleep on their side with their head higher than their feet. If the vomiting is persistent and severe, a paediatrician should be consulted. Most paediatricians recommend a trial period with thickened feeds before a pH recording.

Whooping cough

Vomiting may be so severe in infants with whooping cough that the parents are more worried by the vomiting than the cough. During the first 5 days of the illness (catarrhal phase) there is a short, dry nocturnal cough (Figure 12.6). Later, bouts of 10–20 short coughs occur day and night. The cough is dry and each cough is on the same high note or goes up in a musical scale. The long attack of coughing is followed by a sharp indrawing of breath, which causes the whoop (see page 102). Some children with proved pertussis infection never develop the whoop. Feeding often provokes a spasm of coughing and this may culminate in vomiting. Afterwards there is a short refractory period during which the baby can be fed again without provoking more coughing. In uncomplicated cases there are no abnormal signs in the respiratory system.

Adrenogenital syndrome

The adrenogenital syndrome (salt-losing type) commonly presents with vomiting as the only symptom in boys. The diagnosis is easier in girls, as virilization of the external genitalia will have been noticed at birth (Figure 12.7). Symptoms usually begin between the seventh and tenth days and may be fatal within a few days if extra salt and salt-retaining adrenocorticosteroids are not given. Intravenous fluids are essential. The diagnosis is confirmed by raised plasma 17-hydroxyprogesterone, high plasma potassium and low plasma sodium concentrations. The plasma electrolyte concentrations are normal at birth and pronounced changes may occur suddenly.

Further reading

Rennie JM. (2005) *Robertson's Textbook of Neonatology*, 4th edn. Churchill Livingstone, Edinburgh.

CHAPTER 13

Diarrhoea

OVERVIEW

- The stools of a normal infant vary with age and diet
- The main danger of gastroenteritis is dehydration and electrolyte imbalance
- Oral rehydration should be started at an early stage at home with specific guidance on the volumes to be given and when and how to obtain further advice
- Recently introduced rotavirus vaccines may have a major effect on the prevalence of acute gastroenteritis

Diarrhoea is the passage of loose stools more often than would be expected from the diet and age of the infant. It indicates a change in bowel habit. A stool should be examined personally. A rectal examination is often followed by a fresh stool, which can be examined. When diarrhoea is severe, the stools may be mistaken for urine. When this is a possibility, a urine bag should be placed in position and the infant nursed on a sheet of polyethylene.

The stools of newborn infants vary with their diet. The normal stools of breastfed infants are never formed, may be passed at hourly intervals, may contain mucus and may be green (Figures 13.1 & 13.2). When lactation becomes established between the third and fifth days intestinal hurry is common, resulting in frequent stools. No treatment is needed. Later the stools tend to become less frequent and more pasty and by the age of 3 weeks they may be passed once every 2 or 3 days. In contrast, the normal stools of bottle-fed infants are formed and do not contain fluid or mucus. With certain cow's milk preparations the stools may be dark green, but this has no sinister meaning.

Acute gastroenteritis

Acute gastroenteritis is an acute infection mainly affecting the small intestine that causes diarrhoea with or without vomiting. The main danger is dehydration and electrolyte imbalance, which may develop rapidly, but the infant may also be very infectious for

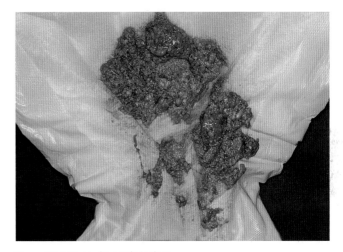

Figure 13.1 Stool of breastfed infant.

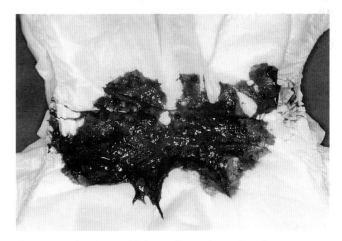

Figure 13.2 Changing stool (mixture of meconium and stool).

other infants in a ward or nursery (Box 13.1). Gastroenteritis is particularly dangerous in infants aged under 2 years.

The early signs of dehydration are often difficult to detect, but recent weight loss is often a valuable indicator. Sunken eyes, inelastic skin and a dry tongue are late signs, but if the infant has not passed urine for several hours severe dehydration is probable. Clinical signs of dehydration are particularly difficult to detect in fat toddlers.

ABC of the First Year, Sixth edition. By B. Valman and R. Thomas. © 2009 Blackwell Publishing, ISBN: 978-1-4051-8037-5.

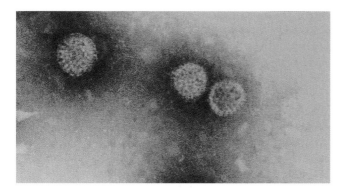

Figure 13.3 Rotavirus.

Table 13.1 Fluid intake in relation to weight.

Baby's weight		Daily fluid intake	
kg	lb	mL	fl. oz
Under 4	Under 9	500	18
4	9	600	21
5	11	750	26
6	13	900	32
7	15	1050	37
8	18	1200	42
9	20	1350	48
Over 10	Over 22	1500	53

The infant must be examined in detail to exclude any other acute infection.

The rotavirus is the most common cause of gastroenteritis in infants and children throughout the world (Figure 13.3). It affects every age group and infection easily spreads throughout a family, although infected adults may have few or no symptoms. Several distinct episodes of diarrhoea can be due to the rotavirus, as there are several serotypes. The incubation period is 24–48 hours and a respiratory illness, including otitis media, precedes the gastrointestinal symptoms in about half the patients. Vomiting, which lasts for 1 to 3 days, is followed by abnormal stools for about 5 days. Treatment is aimed at keeping infants well hydrated until they recover spontaneously. The frequency of the stools is reduced by dietary treatment, but the abnormal consistency of the stools persists for up to a week.

If infants are given an antibiotic early in the illness (for example, when acute otitis media is suspected as the primary diagnosis) the subsequent diarrhoea may be attributed to the antibiotic rather than to the rotavirus infection. Other drugs (for example, iron) may be associated with diarrhoea.

Management

Clinical signs of severe dehydration or the loss of 5% or more of body weight are definite indications for admission. If infants relapse after treatment or social problems prevent them being treated at home they may need to be admitted. Infants who vomit persistently usually need to be admitted, though mild symptoms may be managed at home by giving small volumes of liquid by mouth every hour.

In mild cases the main principle of management is to stop cow's milk and solids and give a glucose or sucrose solution orally. After 24 hours fruit or vegetable purees may be introduced and then other items from the child's normal diet. Cow's milk and cow's milk products are reintroduced gradually after the first 24 hours of

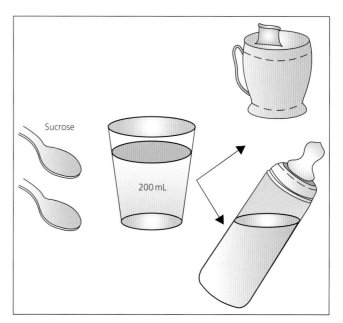

Figure 13.4 Rehydrating fluid for use at home.

treatment. Vomiting may be reduced by giving small volumes of fluid frequently. The child should be allowed to drink as much as he or she wants but needs at least the volume shown in Table 13.1.

Rarely, a breastfed infant has gastroenteritis, but the symptoms are usually mild. The appropriate volume of rehydrating fluid is given by bottle or spoon before each breastfeed for 24 hours and then normal breastfeeding is restarted.

Kaolin should not be prescribed as it deflects the mother's attention from the main treatment. No antibiotics should be given to children with gastroenteritis treated at home.

The ideal oral rehydrating fluid is a glucose–electrolyte mixture, but a 4% sucrose solution is easily available and safe. Single dose sachets of glucose–electrolyte powder are available from pharmacists without prescription, which enable parents to make up the mixture accurately at home. A safe alternative is 4% sucrose solution, which can be made up using 2 level teaspoonfuls of granulated sucrose in 200 mL water (Figure 13.4). It is dangerous to add salt to this mixture.

Box 13.2 **Investigations**

- Stool culture
- ELISA rotavirus stool test
- Urine microscopy and culture
- Plasma sodium, potassium and urea estimations

Box 13.3 **Causes of relapse**

- Failure to follow plan
- Temporary intolerance to cow's milk

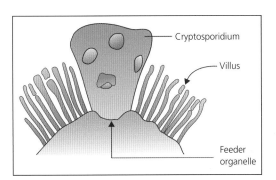

Figure 13.5 *Cryptosporidium* is intracellular, separated from rest of cytoplasm by a feeder organelle.

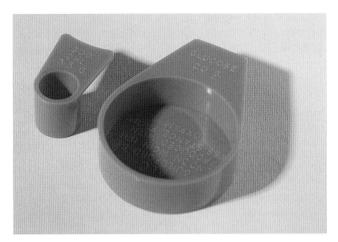

Figure 13.6 Spoons to measure sugar and salt for rehydration fluid.

In severe cases of dehydration or persistent vomiting oral fluids must be replaced with intravenous fluids in infants admitted to hospital. During the next day the fluid requirement should be given as an oral glucose–electrolyte mixture, alternating with full-strength cow's milk formula, and fruit and vegetable purees are introduced. Most children are discharged from hospital on a normal diet within a few days of admission.

The importance of handwashing and food hygiene should be stressed as spread occurs by the faecal–oral or respiratory routes. Infants in hospital with diarrhoea must be barrier nursed in a cubicle, which should ideally be in an annexe to the children's ward.

Investigations (Box 13.2)

Ideally a stool should be sent to the laboratory for detection of pathogens, but this is not necessary for mild cases treated at home. Only a small proportion of children have bacteria such as *Campylobacter*, *Salmonella* or *Shigella* isolated from their stools. *Cryptosporidium*, a protozoon which can be seen by light microscopy, is a common pathogen (Figure 13.5). Most cases of gastroenteritis in children are caused by viruses, usually rotavirus, and can be identified by an ELISA slide test. Blood in the fluid stool suggests the presence of Shiga toxin which may cause haemolytic–uraemic syndrome.

Children needing intravenous fluids should have their plasma electrolyte, bicarbonate and urea concentrations measured urgently.

If two or more infants in a ward or nursery have diarrhoea at the same time cross-infection should be presumed, even if their stool cultures show no pathogens. Stools from all the infants on the ward should be sent for culture and tests for rotavirus. Admissions to the ward may have to be stopped.

Progress

The infant should be reviewed again by the doctor within 24 hours of starting treatment to ensure that the illness is resolving, the infant is not losing too much weight, and the carers understand the management. Severe dehydration can occur within a few hours and it is important to have a specific policy to ensure adequate follow-up visits.

The main cause of relapse or persistent symptoms is failure to follow a plan of treatment (Box 13.3). Social problems may indicate a need for admission to hospital. A few infants aged under 2 years have temporary mucosal damage and are intolerant to cow's milk or other foods. This causes the diarrhoea to persist for longer than 2 weeks and is considered on page 80.

Gastroenteritis in developing countries

In developing countries continuing breastfeeding during attacks of gastroenteritis may be essential for survival. Although infants who are completely breastfed rarely have severe gastroenteritis, weaning foods made up with water may infect a breastfed infant. These infants can be managed by continuing the breastfeeding and supplementing the fluid intake to prevent dehydration until the infant spontaneously recovers. Supplements may be given by mouth in mild cases and intravenously in severe cases. An easier method is to give them by continuous intragastric infusion, for which the fluid does not have to be sterile.

Oral rehydrating fluids can be made up using specially designed spoons to measure the sugar and salt (Figure 13.6). Mothers and older siblings can be taught to use this mixture at the beginning of an episode of diarrhoea rather than wait until the child is dehydrated. Simple slogans such as 'a cup of fluid for every stool' are effective.

Further reading

Elliott EJ. (2007) Acute gastroenteritis in children. *British Medical Journal* 334: 35–40.

CHAPTER 14

Mother–Infant Attachment

OVERVIEW

- Mothers and infants need to be close physically for optimal development of the infant
- The newborn infant can see, hear, taste and smell, and communication between mother and infant promotes attachment
- Separation for a short period, although distressing to the mother, has no permanent detrimental effect on the infant

There is no specific sensitive period immediately after delivery that is the only time that emotional attachment can form. Any important effects of separation do not persist beyond days or weeks after reunion. Parents who have read obsolete publications may need reassurance that early separation is not followed by permanent damage to mother–infant relationships. A comparison of preterm and term babies indicated that parents find the behaviour of preterm babies less predictable and more frustrating. Though frequent and sustained contact with a sick or preterm baby may increase the degree of parental anxiety, this anxiety induces a feeling of involvement in the care of their baby.

A biological need

Mothers and infants need a close attachment to give the infant the degree of security necessary for optimal emotional and physical development.

Most mothers have strong maternal feelings, which enable them to achieve a firm bond of affection with their babies without difficulty, even after an initial period of separation. The strength of their maternal feelings probably depends on the quality of mothering they received in infancy (Figure 14.3).

In contrast, a mother may be unable to achieve this attachment without close contact with her baby and even then, it may take a few days before the baby appears to her to be an individual and her own. Failure to form a normal attachment probably accounts for the higher incidence of 'battered babies' among preterm infants

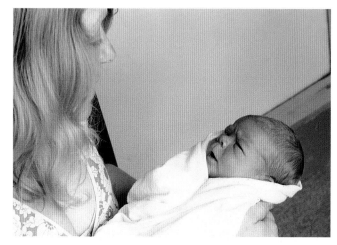

Figure 14.1 A newborn infant looking at mother.

and among the infants of mothers who were themselves deprived of maternal care.

Forming an attachment

Attachment occurs in five main ways (Figure 14.2). Firstly, infants can follow the mother's eyes immediately after birth and this eye to eye contact is an important factor (Figure 14.1).

Secondly, a mother left with her naked infant touches each part of the baby's body with her fingertips.

Thirdly, during the first few days after delivery mothers often appear to overprotect their infants and become overanxious about crying and minor difficulties, such as those of feeding.

Fourthly, even in the first days of life babies mimic the facial expressions of others and can, for example, put out their tongues at them, providing 'feedback'.

Lastly, physical contact during breastfeeding and the presence of the baby next to the mother throughout the entire 24 hours also promote attachment.

Separation

Separation is sometimes unavoidable if, for example, the infant has to be transferred to another unit for surgery (Figure 14.4) or the mother is receiving heavy sedation for hypertension. The mother is

ABC of the First Year, Sixth edition. By B. Valman and R. Thomas. © 2009 Blackwell Publishing, ISBN: 978-1-4051-8037-5.

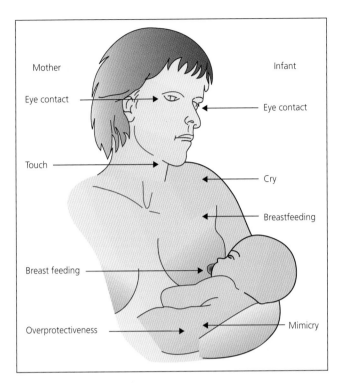

Figure 14.2 Factors in attachment.

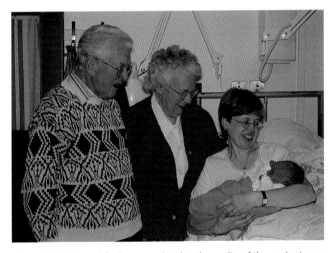

Figure 14.3 Maternal feelings are related to the quality of the mother's own mothering.

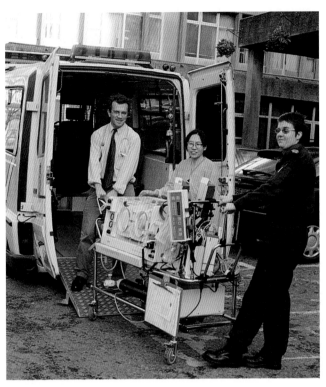

Figure 14.4 Separation may be necessary for medical reasons.

equally separated from her child when she is severely depressed, but this may not appear so obvious.

In the past many babies were separated from their mothers for reasons that would not now be acceptable. Owing to doctors' anxiety, infants with jaundice were admitted to special care units even though they needed no special care. The number of nursing staff available on individual maternity wards will determine whether it is safe for babies to remain with their mothers, but no infant should be separated from his or her mother without good reason.

A postnatal ward should be staffed with midwives who have special experience in nursing babies of low birthweight. This allows babies needing tube feeding and other forms of special care to remain with their mothers and avoids the separation resulting

from admission to the neonatal unit. The care of healthy but low birthweight infants in the same environment as their mothers is called transitional care to indicate that they need more support than normal term infants.

Difficulty in forming attachments

Some aspects of the history may suggest that a mother may have difficulty in forming an attachment to her infant and will need special help from nursing and medical staff. Particularly vulnerable are mothers who had poor maternal care in their own childhood, who have had a request for an abortion rejected or who have not decided whether they want the infant to be adopted. If a previous infant was stillborn or died in the neonatal period or a close relative has recently died, help may also be needed. Special attention should be given to a mother under 17 years of age.

When the baby is born, the mother may refuse to handle or feed him or her and be more concerned with her own minor symptoms than the infant's care. She may feel detached and the infant's problems may appear to her to be more serious than they are. Similar symptoms may be the first indication of a severe depression in the mother and she may need psychiatric help (Figure 14.5).

Encouraging attachment

To encourage attachment the principle is to avoid unnecessary separation. Unless infants require special nursing they should be given to their mothers in the labour room, even if an abnormality such as Down syndrome is present. Newborn infants are able to feed moments after birth even if the mother has received sedation

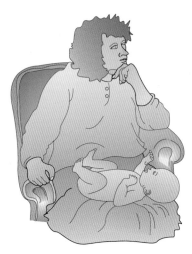

Figure 14.5 Detachment due to depression.

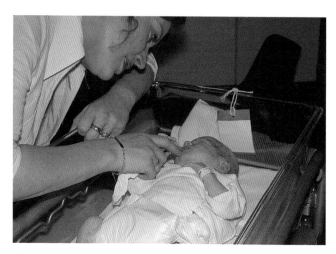

Figure 14.7 Talking to and touching the baby.

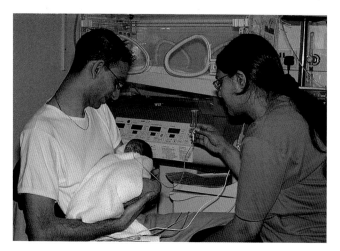

Figure 14.6 Parents should be encouraged to care for their infant in the neonatal unit.

and the mother should be encouraged to put the baby to her breast if she intends to breastfeed. Infants should remain with the mother throughout the 24 hours of the day and be taken out at night only if they continually disturb the other mothers in the room. Breastfeeding should be actively encouraged, though this may take time and perseverance by both mothers and nursing staff. Mothers of preterm infants should be encouraged to express their milk and thus feel that they are actively contributing to the infant's welfare.

In neonatal units the atmosphere should make parents feel that they are welcome at any time and they should be encouraged to look at, touch, change, feed and later breastfeed their infants (Figure 14.6). When parents are about to visit a very sick infant the reasons for the use of special apparatus should be explained beforehand. A mother can usually visit her infant in the neonatal unit the day after a caesarean section by being wheeled in a chair.

If a mother fails to visit her infant for long periods after she has been discharged, an inquiry should be made as to whether any remediable reason, such as lack of transport, is responsible.

Before the infant is discharged from the unit the mother should remain with her infant in a room on the unit for at least 24 hours,

but longer if possible. This gives her an opportunity to gain confidence in her ability to cope with her baby, who recently appeared to be so fragile and needing expert nursing care to survive.

What the newborn baby can do

Some parents, especially those having their first baby, believe that newborn babies are blind until they are 6 weeks old. It is not surprising that these parents treat their babies like inanimate dolls and feel ashamed when an unexpected visitor catches them talking to the baby. The normal newborn infant can see, hear and appreciate pain immediately after birth, even if the mother has received heavy sedation. During the hour after birth the infant is often wide awake, looking round for a feed before going to sleep for a few hours (Figure 14.7).

The distance between the eyes of the mother and the infant when the mother is breastfeeding is the distance at which infants can best focus on an object. This eye-to-eye contact provides the first means of communication between mother and infant and is probably the reason why mothers find that covering the infant's eyes during phototherapy disturbs them. Mothers of blind infants have difficulty in feeling close to their infants. Newborn infants will become alert, frown, and gradually try to focus on a red object dangled about 30 cm before them. They stare intently at the object and will follow it with short jerking movements of the eyes if it is moved slowly from side to side (Figure 14.8). Infants are also sensitive to the intensity of light and will shut their eyes tightly and keep them shut if bright light is turned on. They can discriminate shapes and patterns and the arrangements of lines from birth. They prefer patterns to dull or bright solid colours, and look longer at stripes and angles than at circular patterns.

Newborn infants can hear. They respond to sound by blinking, jerking their limbs, or drawing in breath. They may stop feeding. Mothers often speak to their infants in a high-pitched voice and infants respond more consistently to their mother's than their father's voice. An infant of 3 days of age shows preference for sweet and dislike of bitter-flavoured fluid. At about the same age he or she can differentiate smells and distinguish between his or her own mother's and other mothers' breast pads.

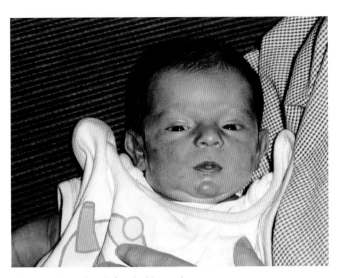

Figure 14.8 Newborn infant looking at the camera.

Analysis of sound films shows that both listener and speaker are moving in time to the words of the speaker, creating a type of dance. For example, as the speaker pauses for breath or accentuates a syllable, the infant may raise an eyebrow or lower a foot. The mother notices these changes and this may encourage her to continue speaking. At a few weeks or even a few days after birth the infant may mimic gestures such as tongue protrusion, lip protrusion or opening the mouth.

If the doctor talks to babies while examining them, parents will not feel foolish when they do it themselves.

Further reading

Barker P. (2004) *Basic Child Psychiatry*, 5th edn. Blackwell Publishing, Oxford.

CHAPTER 15

Growth and Growth Charts

OVERVIEW

- Most infants have a similar centile at birth for weight and head circumference, and remain on the same centiles
- Where one parent is relatively tall or short, the infant may change centiles for both weight and head circumference during the first year
- Plotting serial measurements on a chart indicates whether the infant is growing normally, becoming overweight or failing to thrive

Weight and head circumference

The size of the normal infant at birth is determined mainly by the mother's size. The greatest changes to adjust for other hereditary factors take place during the first 3 months of life. Although children tend to attain a stature between those of their parents, some children take after one parent or grandparent, or an even more remote member of the family. All these children are perfectly healthy. It may be difficult to distinguish these normal adjustments of growth from disease, especially during the first few months of life. Growth charts are therefore essential for diagnosis during this period and helpful in discussions with parents. The growth charts in this chapter have been devised to illustrate the text and were not drawn from observed measurements.

Length (or height) is difficult to measure accurately in a very young baby and for some years we have used the head circumference as a reference measurement for comparison with the weight. The use of the head circumference in this way is valuable only in the first 2 years of life. The head circumference is measured round the occipitofrontal circumference (the largest circumference), which should be determined with a disposable paper tape measure (Figure 15.1). Linen tape measures stretch and produce inaccurate results.

Normal growth and small normal infants

An infant usually has a similar centile at birth for both head circumference and weight. Children of large parents tend to be

ABC of the First Year, Sixth edition. By B. Valman and R. Thomas. © 2009 Blackwell Publishing, ISBN: 978-1-4051-8037-5.

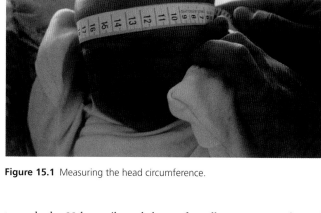

Figure 15.1 Measuring the head circumference.

towards the 98th centile and those of small parents near the 2nd centile. Most of these children remain on the same centiles for the rest of their lives. Plotting these measurements on a Chart in routine clinics helps to confirm that the child is receiving adequate food and is growing normally.

One of the most common problems in paediatric outpatient clinics is short parents who think that their infant does not eat enough. Plotting growth measurements on a chart from measurements already recorded at the local clinic confirms to the doctor and the parents that the child is normal and that the child's final size will be similar to that of the parents (Chart A). Charts are better than cards for recording growth (Figure 15.2).

Taking after father or mother

Some children are more similar to one parent than the other in final size. If only their weights are recorded, they may appear to be either failing to thrive if the father is small (Chart B) or gaining weight excessively if the father is tall (Chart C). If both weight and head circumference are plotted on a chart, the weight centile line and head circumference centile line can be seen to be running in parallel. In other words, the whole of the child's size is approaching that of a particular parent.

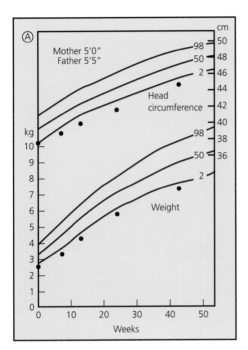

Chart A Small normal infant.

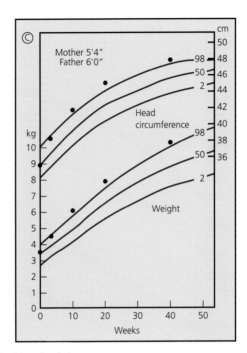

Chart C Taking after father.

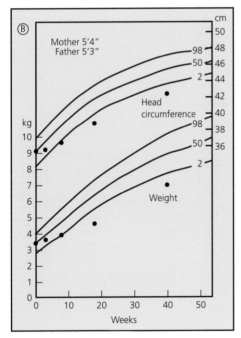

Chart B Taking after father.

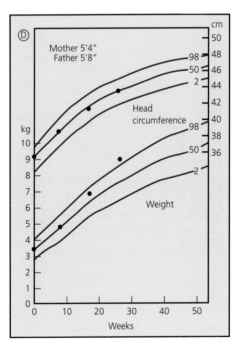

Chart D Obesity.

Getting fat

Growth charts give an early warning of obesity. Chart D shows that at the age of 20 weeks this child's weight centile started deviating upwards although the head circumference centile remained the same. If the mother had been shown the growth chart at the age of 20 weeks she might have been able to prevent the phenomenon seen at 30 weeks.

The standard growth charts are based on data collected when the majority of babies were fed with cow's milk preparations. Some normal breastfed babies gain weight rapidly in the first 10 weeks and then more slowly during the subsequent 20 weeks

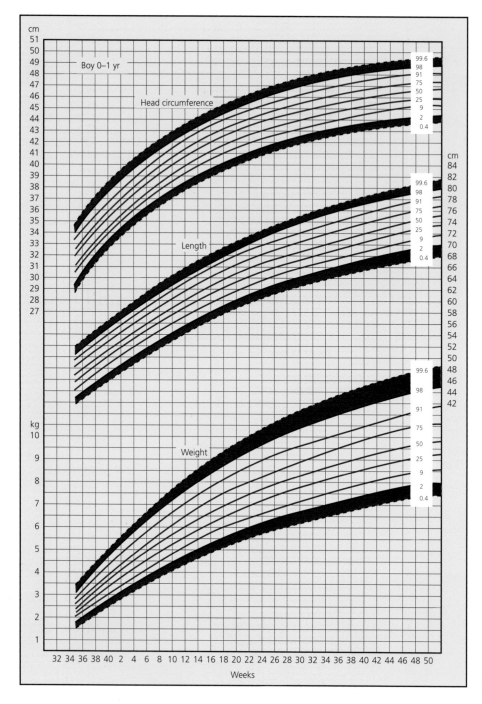

Figure 15.2 Growth chart.

(Chart E). This is a normal growth pattern and is not an indication of obesity.

Poor lactation and failure to thrive

The increased incidence of breastfeeding has resulted in a few infants receiving insufficient milk because their mothers have not recognized poor lactation. This can be detected at an early stage by weighing infants regularly, although normal breastfed infants may not regain their birthweights before the age of 2 weeks. The onset of full lactation is extremely variable and this must be taken into account when considering the adequacy of weight gain (Chart F). Plotting the infant's weight on a growth chart is the first investigation required to diagnose whether failure to thrive is present and also to give a presumptive diagnosis of the cause (Chart G).

Preterm

When preterm infants reach home, they may gain weight rapidly, when they will cross the centile lines for both weight and head circumference in parallel (Chart H). Preterm infants may have a

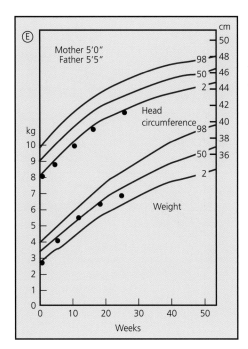

Chart E Normal breastfed infant.

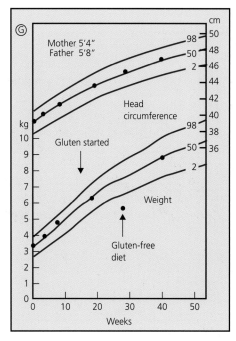

Chart G Coeliac disease.

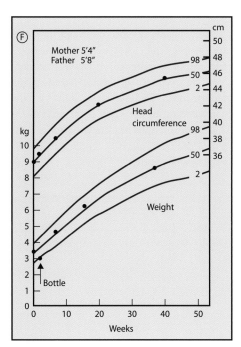

Chart F Poor lactation.

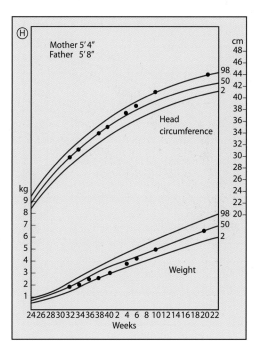

Chart H Catch-up growth in preterm infant.

relatively large head measurement because of the head's discoid shape, but continuing growth on the same centile line shows that the head is normal. Babies of extremely low gestational age, especially below 26 weeks, with chronic lung disease may continue to grow poorly despite feeding well.

Infants whose growth *in utero* has been restricted due to poor nutrition related to placental function may have catch-up growth (Chart H) or may continue to grow poorly postnatally (Chart I).

Infant of diabetic mother

The infant of the diabetic mother may be grossly obese at birth but slims down within a few months of birth (Chart J). These infants may not gain any weight at all for the first 2 months of life and the mother may be accused of underfeeding the infant.

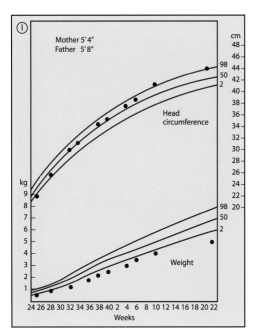

Chart I Poor weight gain and discoid head in preterm infant.

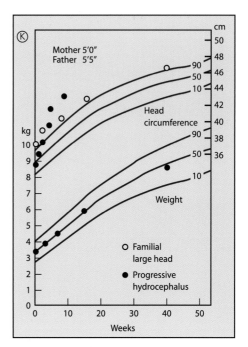

Chart K Progressive hydrocephalus.

Progressive hydrocephalus

Progressive hydrocephalus can be confirmed by showing a head circumference centile that progressively increases while the weight centile shows no change (Chart K). It may occur in association with intraventricular haemorrhage in preterm infants or myelomeningocoele. Hydrocephalus can be confirmed by ultrasound examination of the brain if the anterior fontanelle is still open. This condition must be differentiated from familial large head, where the head circumference centile remains constant and is parallel to the weight centile.

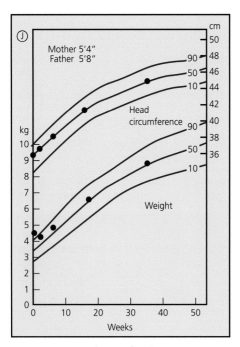

Chart J Infant of diabetic mother.

CHAPTER 16

Feeding and Feeding Problems

OVERVIEW

- Human milk has a unique composition and contains protective factors against infection
- Complementary feeding may be needed if there is insufficient breast milk
- Some mothers do not want to breastfeed and should not be put under pressure to change
- Problems with feeding can be identified by taking a simple history and weighing the infant

The national infant feeding survey in 2005 showed that 78% of mothers in England breastfed their babies initially and this had increased by 6% on the previous survey in 2000. There has been a steady increase in breastfeeding since 1990. The highest incidences of breastfeeding were found among mothers from managerial and professional occupations, those with the highest educational levels, those aged 30 years or more and first-time mothers. Between 2000 and 2005 breastfeeding rates across the UK increased by a greater degree among mothers of second or later babies compared with mothers of first-time babies. At 6 weeks 42% of mothers were still breastfeeding and at 6 months 21%. The most common reason given by mothers for breastfeeding was that it was best for the baby's health and for bottle feeding that it allowed others to feed the baby.

Full-term infants usually regain their birthweight between the seventh and tenth day, and thereafter the infant should gain about 20–40 g/day for the next 100 days. Unmodified milk ('doorstep' milk) should not be given until after the age of 1 year and should be accompanied by vitamin supplements, particularly vitamin D, until the age of 4 years. Progress on a growth chart is the best guide to ensuring that an infant is receiving the correct amount of milk (Figure 16.1).

Breastfeeding

Breastfeeding should be encouraged for several reasons (Figure 16.2). Firstly, the fat and protein of human milk are more completely

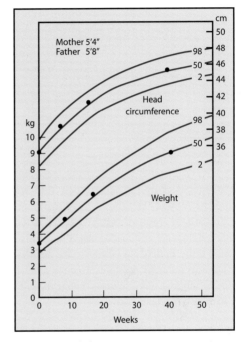

Figure 16.1 Normal growth chart.

absorbed than those of cow's milk. The composition of human milk varies during a feed and these subtle changes cannot be mimicked by cow's milk preparations. The significance of these changes is unknown but may be related to the control of intake by appetite.

Secondly, the fat composition and therefore the fatty acid composition of breast milk vary during a feed, these changes cannot be replaced exactly by cow's milk preparations and the differences in body composition resulting from these different milks may have a long-term effect.

Thirdly, human milk contains antibodies and iron binding protein (lactoferrin) which may protect the infant against infections. Gastroenteritis is rare in breastfed infants.

Breastfeeding also plays an important part in mother–infant attachment. If the mother is encouraged during the antenatal period to expect to be able to breastfeed her baby and eventually to enjoy it, she is likely to accept early difficulties with patience and understanding. The close contact and intimacy, and often supreme

ABC of the First Year, Sixth edition. By B. Valman and R. Thomas. © 2009 Blackwell Publishing, ISBN: 978-1-4051-8037-5.

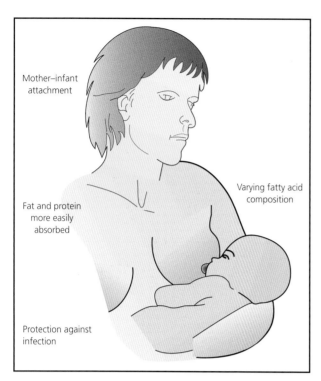

Figure 16.2 Advantages of breastfeeding.

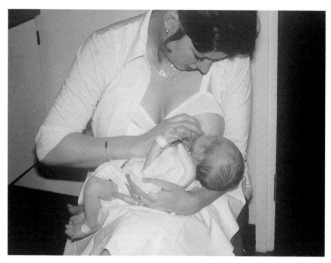

Figure 16.3 Breastfeeding.

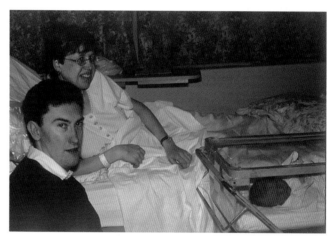

Figure 16.4 Rooming in.

enjoyment, of breastfeeding provide the best 'feedback' between the baby and the mother. The mother's intimate personal relationship with her baby is something that she has to work out for herself. Many feel insecure and inadequate at first and are only too glad to change to bottle feeding whenever the slightest difficulty arises. The attendant should resist such requests and instead use sympathy, understanding and skill to encourage the mother to gain confidence in breastfeeding her baby.

Latching to the breast

The sensation of the nipple against the palate stimulates the baby to suck. Placing the baby in the correct position encourages successful feeding and avoids damage to the nipple. The baby's chin must drive into the breast to enable the nipple to reach the palate, so the baby needs to put his or her head back and up. If the baby's head becomes too flexed, the nipple touches the lower jaw and the tongue and the nose is too close to the breast. Helping the chin to thrust forwards and the head to tilt back is hindered by pressure on the back of the head but improved by supporting the baby's back at shoulder level, with the baby facing the mother, chest to chest.

Rooming in

A normal infant is put to the breast for a few minutes at each side either immediately or a few hours after birth (Figure 16.3). Only a small amount of colostrum is obtained but sucking by the infant stimulates the production of more milk. Some infants are reluctant to take the nipple initially and the mother needs strong reassurance that this is common.

During the first week, and probably later, most of the feed is obtained within 4 minutes in some babies. Thus the length of time that the baby is on the breast bears little relation to the amount of

milk received by the infant. Some infants take a shorter time and others a longer time to take a full feed.

The most satisfactory method of breastfeeding is 'on demand'. Babies commonly feed every 2 or 3 hours during the first few weeks and these frequent feeds are a powerful stimulus to lactation. This is the main advantage of rooming in, where the infant's cot is by the side of the mother's bed and she can pick her baby up and feed them when they cry (Figure 16.4). Mothers should be encouraged to do this. Infants initially fed on demand usually settle down to a regular schedule after a few weeks. Most breastfed infants feed 3-hourly rather than 4-hourly.

Complementary feeding

If the infant is crying frequently, despite breastfeeding on demand, there is a possibility that the infant is receiving insufficient milk from the breast. If the feed is deficient, putting the baby to the breast more frequently may stimulate increased lactation in the early days. If this approach is not effective, the deficit may be made up with a complementary feed given after feeding from both breasts. Fortunately, a well nourished full-term infant can tolerate a degree of underfeeding without harm for a few days, but progressive weight loss or failure to regain the birthweight by the 10th day are indications for complementary feeding. The increasing incidence of breastfeeding has been accompanied by a few infants who become dehydrated and lethargic and have hyperbilirubinaemia. These problems could be avoided if new mothers are given appropriate advice and support when establishing breastfeeding in the first few days after birth.

The feel of a teat is different from that of the breast but it is controversial whether a baby will stop breastfeeding if offered a bottle. Most infants continue to feed by both methods. If a mother does not wish to give the baby a bottle, complementary feeds can be given with a syringe or spoon. Other options are a small cup or a reservoir of milk with a small tube, which drips milk inside a nipple shield while the infant is breastfeeding. Complementary feeding may be needed for a few weeks until adequate milk is produced from the breasts and can be withdrawn gradually. Previous fears of early sensitization to cow's milk, even if given in small amounts, are now considered to be based on less secure scientific evidence.

Contraindications to breastfeeding

There are few contraindications to breastfeeding (Box 16.1). Some women have a revulsion to the idea and it would be a mistake to try to persuade them. Psychiatric illness in the mother may be aggravated if the baby is taken off the breast. Severely cracked nipple causing maternal discomfort is a temporary contraindication to feeding from the affected breast, but the milk should be expressed with a pump. Feeding should continue from a breast with acute mastitis while the mother is receiving an antibiotic; it should also continue if the nipple is only mildly cracked.

No drugs should be taken by a lactating mother unless there are strong clinical indications. Most drugs that are essential for the mother are secreted in the milk in insignificant amounts, so breastfeeding should not be stopped unless there is a special reason. Antibiotics are excreted in minute amounts in the milk but there is the theoretical possibility of sensitizing the infant. Warfarin, senna, sodium valproate, phenytoin, steroids, antacids and occasional doses of paracetamol pass into the milk in unimportant amounts. Kaolin is not absorbed by the mother. Oestrogens in oral contraceptives may reduce lactation, but the progesterone-only pill is an effective contraceptive and has no effect on lactation. A mother receiving carbimazole may continue to breastfeed provided that the infant's plasma thyroxine concentration is monitored.

Mothers receiving radioactive antithyroid treatment or cytotoxic drugs should not breastfeed. Lithium given to the mother may cause hypotonia, hypothermia and episodes of cyanosis in a breastfed infant.

Problems with breastfeeding

On the fourth or fifth day, when there is a plentiful supply of breast milk, the infant may take up to eight feeds or more a day.

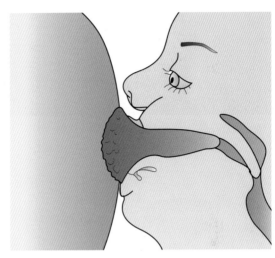

Figure 16.5 Good placement of the nipple in the infant's mouth.

Intestinal hurry and frequent loose green stools are common at this stage (Box 16.2). Conversely, some normal breastfed infants pass stools only once a week when they reach the age of a few weeks, and this also requires no treatment.

Cracked nipple is usually due to misplacement of the infant on the nipple so that the whole of the pigmented area is not in the infant's mouth (Figure 16.5). Pulling the infant off the breast abruptly is another cause. If the nipple is slightly cracked, breastfeeding should continue with advice on latching to the breast. If the crack is severe, the infant should be taken off that breast for a day or so and a bland ointment, such as lanolin, placed on the nipple every few hours. A fissure of the nipple occurring after the first few weeks is often aggravated by thrush infection of the baby's mouth and the mother's nipple. It is best treated in both mother and infant with miconazole or nystatin gel until 4 days after it appears to be clear.

In acute mastitis there is fever, pain, flushing, induration in one breast and enlarged axillary lymph nodes. Flucloxacillin or erythromycin is given to the mother for at least a week and feeding continues from both breasts. Fluctuation in the indurated area indicates that an abscess is present and the need for surgical incision.

Feeding on demand usually prevents maternal breast engorgement, which can occur towards the end of the first week of the baby's life. This is alleviated by expression after feeding, preferably with a pump (Figure 16.6). If engorgement has already occurred the help of an experienced midwife is necessary.

During the first feed of the morning milk may spurt quickly from the breast and a ravenous infant may swallow excessive air, which may be regurgitated later with milk. This is often

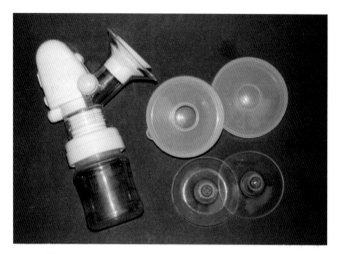

Figure 16.6 Breast pump.

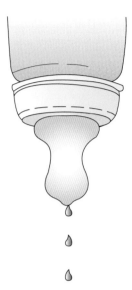

Figure 16.8 Drops should follow each other quickly.

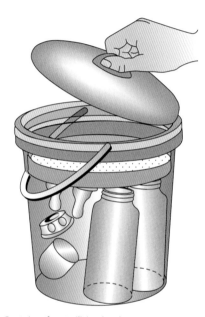

Figure 16.7 Container for sterilizing bottles.

the best method in hospitals. Another method is steam in a special microwave oven kit. Teats should be well washed before sterilization.

The size of the hole in the teat should allow individual drops of milk to follow each other quickly when the bottle is inverted, and this should be checked each week (Figure 16.8).

'On demand' feeding

Feeds are usually given 'on demand' or 3- or 4-hourly. Most infants need to be fed every 3 hours. The milk must not be made up to a stronger concentration than that recommended on the packet. Few babies can manage without a night feed for the first few months.

A normal full-term infant receives 30 mL of milk per kg body weight during the first day of feeding by bottle. Feeds should be increased by 20 mL/kg each day until a maximum of 150 mL/kg is reached on the seventh day of feeding. Underfeeding causes small amounts of green mucus to be passed frequently, but this is more likely to be found with breastfed than with bottle-fed infants.

Problems with bottle feeding

If the hole in the teat is too small the infant may swallow excessive air during the feed and regurgitate it later with milk, accompanied by bouts of crying. It is valuable to observe the rate at which the drops of milk are formed when the infant's bottle is inverted. The drops should follow each other quickly but there should not be a continuous stream. If the hole is too small it may be made larger with a hot needle. If the hole is too large, infants may also swallow excessive air as they gulp to avoid choking.

By taking a careful history it is usually possible to determine the likely cause of any symptoms. If growth is poor, infants need more frequent or larger feeds. If the weather is hot and infants are not receiving extra water, they may be thirsty and should have additional water. Mothers tend to use gripe water as a panacea, not realising that it contains bicarbonate, which produces carbon dioxide gas when it reacts with gastric acid in the stomach.

accompanied by severe crying. It can be alleviated by manual expression of the first 30 mL of milk, which can be given to the infant later if necessary.

Bottle feeding

All the cow's milk preparations available in the UK have sodium and protein concentrations similar to those of human milk. The powder should be measured accurately, avoiding heaped or packed scoops. The instructions on each packet must be followed. Ready to feed bottles are used in most obstetric units.

If feeds are made up for a 24-hour period they should be cooled and stored in the refrigerator. After use, bottles and teats should be washed in tap water with a brush, or in a dishwasher at 65°C, and then sterilized. Bottles can be sterilized in dilute hypochlorite solution (Figure 16.7), but processing in an autoclave is

Reluctance to feed

In an infant who has fed normally before, reluctance to feed may be a dangerous symptom. It may be due to any severe disease, such as congenital heart disease, or a lower respiratory tract infection. On the other hand, when an infant has a mild upper respiratory tract infection the nose may become blocked with mucus making it difficult for the baby to feed. Thrush produces white plaques on the buccal mucosa and tongue, which become sore. It can be treated by a course of oral nystatin drops or miconazole oral gel.

Further reading

Royal College of Midwives. (2002) *Successful Breastfeeding.* Churchill Livingstone, London.

CHAPTER 17

Failure to Thrive

OVERVIEW

- Failure to thrive is an abnormally low rate of weight gain
- It is detected by plotting serial measurements of weight and head circumference on a growth chart
- The main causes are deficient intake of food, which may be due to social or psychiatric factors, and excessive loss from malabsorption

Mothers become anxious if their infants do not gain weight at the rate that they expect. The majority of these babies are perfectly healthy but their parents' expectations are too high. Initially, it is essential to determine whether the baby is gaining weight normally (Box 17.1). If weight gain is abnormal, failure to thrive is present and a cause should be sought. Some of the material in this chapter is also found in Chapter 15.

Normal weight gain

Small parents
An infant usually has a similar centile at birth for both head circumference and weight. Children of large parents tend to be towards the 98th centile and those of small parents near the 2nd centile. Most of these children remain on the same centiles for the rest of their lives. Plotting these measurements on a chart helps to confirm that children are receiving adequate food and are growing normally. A common problem is the infant of short parents who consider that their child does not eat enough (Chart A). Plotting growth measurements on a chart from measurements already recorded in the personal child health record, held by the parents, confirms to the doctor and the parents that the child is normal

Box 17.1 **Order of priorities**

- Is the weight gain normal?
- If not, what is the cause?

ABC of the First Year, Sixth edition. By B. Valman and R. Thomas. © 2009 Blackwell Publishing, ISBN: 978-1-4051-8037-5.

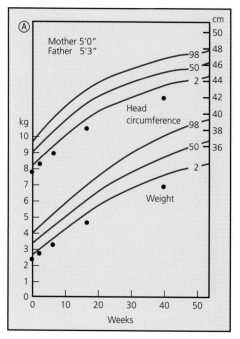

Chart A Normal infant of small parents.

and that his or her final size will be similar to that of the parents. Charts are better than lists of measurements for seeing the trends in growth.

Taking after father or mother
Some children are more similar to one parent than the other in final size. If only their weight is recorded they may appear to be either failing to thrive if the father is small (Chart B) or gaining weight excessively if the father is tall (Chart C). If both weight and head circumference are plotted on a chart, the weight centile line and head circumference centile line can be seen to be running in parallel. In other words, the whole of the child's size is approaching that of a particular parent.

Low birthweight
Infants who are of low birthweight may have been born early (preterm) or have experienced intrauterine malnutrition or both. Although some of them have a period of 'catch-up' growth during the first few months of life, others remain below the 2nd centile

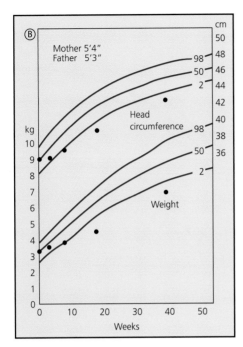

Chart B Taking after father.

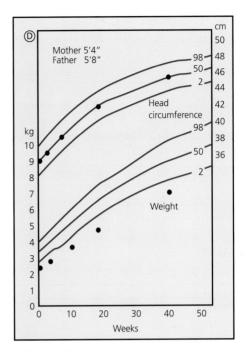

Chart D Low birthweight.

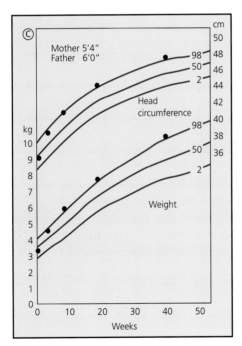

Chart C Taking after father.

for the whole of their lives. This is considered to be related to the intrauterine malnutrition (see Chart D).

Physical causes of failure to thrive

A progressive fall in the weight centile with a constant head circumference centile is the best confirmation of failure to thrive. Measurements on a single occasion may show a weight centile that is below the head circumference and length centile, but these

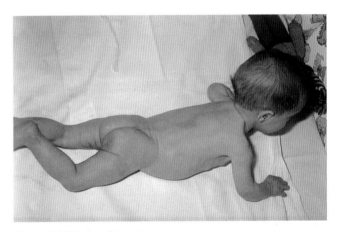

Figure 17.1 Wasting of buttocks.

findings may be present in a normal baby whose family has a body shape that is slightly different from the majority. The plotting of serial measurements on a growth chart before starting to take a history often shortens that process.

Deficient intake of food or excessive loss from malabsorption or metabolic disease cause failure to thrive. Psychiatric and social problems, which are the predominant factor in the majority of the infants with failure to thrive in this country, probably reduce the food intake.

A detailed history is taken, paying particular attention to the family history, birth, feeding and maternal anxieties. Details of any vomiting, diarrhoea or abdominal distension are noted. The complete examination includes an assessment of developmental age and evidence of wasting, particularly of the inner aspects of the thighs and buttocks (Figures 17.1 & 17.2).

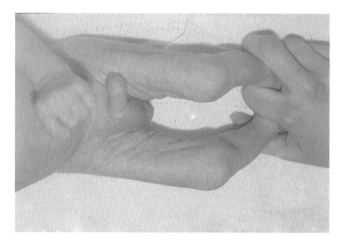

Figure 17.2 Wasting of thighs.

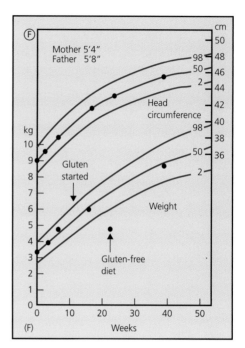

Chart F Coeliac disease.

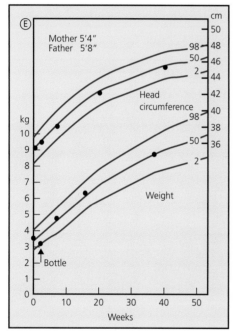

Chart E Poor lactation.

Deficient intake

Poor lactation. The high incidence of breastfeeding in some areas has resulted in a few infants receiving insufficient milk as a result of their mothers' not recognizing poor lactation. This can be detected at an early stage by weighing infants regularly (see Chart E), although normal breastfed infants may not regain their birthweight before the age of 2 weeks. The onset of full lactation is extremely variable and this must be taken into account when considering the adequacy of weight gain (see Chapter 16).

Problems with bottle feeding. Poor tuition may result in deficient milk intake (see Chapter 16).

Cerebral palsy. Infants with cerebral palsy may present with slow feeding and resulting poor milk intake before changes in the motor function in the limbs can be detected. These infants will usually have some evidence of developmental delay.

Congenital heart disease. There may be deficient milk intake due to slow feeding and there is also a high metabolic rate. Central cyanosis, a murmur, or both are usually present.

Urinary infection. A clean-catch urine specimen examined promptly in the laboratory is essential for this diagnosis.

Excessive loss

Gastro-oesophageal reflux. Persistent vomiting from birth may result in failure to thrive if the infant does not take in additional milk to compensate for the loss (see page 59).

Congenital pyloric stenosis. This condition may present at any time before the age of 3 months. It should be considered in any baby less than that age who vomits persistently (see page 58).

Malabsorption. In this country the main causes of malabsorption are cow's milk protein intolerance, cystic fibrosis and coeliac disease (see Chart F). These conditions all cause loose stools that are more frequent than normal, but this may not be recognized by a mother with a first child. A detailed history of bowel function should be taken and personal examination of the stool may be helpful.

Diabetes mellitus. This can be excluded by a negative multistix test for glucose in the urine.

Psychiatric and social factors in failure to thrive

A physical cause for failure to thrive may be present in a family with psychiatric and social problems and therefore a physical cause must be excluded for all infants. The exclusion of a physical cause is often helpful in persuading the parents to accept that psychiatric or social factors are the main reason for the problem. Features in the history that may suggest this possibility include maternal depression, marital discord or a disorganized household. Maternal food preferences may result in the exclusion of certain foods such as cow's milk from the diet without reason and without adequate supervision, and may result in a deficient energy intake.

There are more subtle ways in which maternal emotional factors may affect the infant. The mother may be depressed and tense, and this anxiety is transmitted to the child, who does not feed. The mother then reacts by removing the food. In other families the child may be intrinsically less responsive than the average child to food and this may affect the mother's response to the child at mealtimes. In both these examples the amount of food taken by the child falls to a plateau where the infant appears to be satisfied with the amount given. Another possibility is that the mother keeps to a diet herself as she either is, or perceives herself to be, overweight and also gives a diet to the infant in a similar way.

Some infants are deliberately underfed as part of child abuse. Normal weight gain occurs when the child is fostered.

Effective management of infants with this diagnosis requires a team approach involving a health visitor, the family doctor, a child psychiatrist and paediatrician. Regular advice from a health visitor or dietician often improves the rate of weight gain.

Investigations

Specific investigations are indicated by the history and examination given above, but if there are no pointers to the diagnosis the following investigations are performed: multistix urine test for glucose, full blood count, sweat test, urine microscopy and culture, and plasma creatinine.

Further reading

Valman HB. (2008) *ABC of One to Seven*, 5th edn. Blackwell Publishing, Oxford.

CHAPTER 18

Weaning

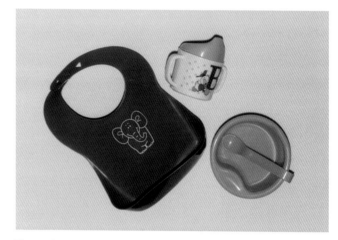

Figure 18.1 Equipment for weaning.

Weaning is the process of getting babies used to eating foods other than milk, and using a spoon and cup. For the first 6 months of life babies will need only milk and additional drinks of boiled water. New foods should start to be introduced at about 6 months. If solid foods are introduced too early babies may become too fat; if they are introduced too late, after 7 months, there may be problems with chewing. Once introduced, solid foods should be given regularly and in gradually increasing quantities. As the amount of solid food increases, the number or size of milk feeds should decrease.

In countries where commercially produced infant cow's milk preparations are safe and affordable, they should be used for the first year of life. Advantages are that the protein and calcium concentrations and vitamin content are more appropriate for babies than unmodified cow's milk.

Mothers need a small, wide plastic teaspoon with no sharp edges, a small plastic cup or bowl, a feeding beaker, and a cotton or plastic-backed cloth bib (Figure 18.1). When babies are 6 months old it is not necessary to sterilize equipment for weaning. Bottles and teats should be sterilized until a beaker or cup is used, and that should be introduced at about this age.

Firstly, babies have to be taught to take food from the spoon rather than just sucking (Figure 18.2). As solids are increased, the volume of milk should be reduced. The baby should also be given plenty to drink to replace the milk; at least 100–150 mL of cooled boiled water each day. Diluted fruit juices are not recommended. Most fruit squashes are unsuitable for babies.

6 months (Box 18.1)

At 6 months babies will usually be having breast or bottle feeds at 6–8 am, 10 am, 2 pm, 6 pm and 10 pm. Solid foods should be introduced to babies before the mid-morning or lunchtime feed – usually a baby cereal or a fruit or vegetable purée.

Mothers should start by using a cereal made from rice and should mix half to one teaspoon of cereal with 1–2 tablespoonfuls of breast milk, infant formula, or water; it should be given to the baby from the spoon. Sugar, honey or salt should not be added. Wheat-based cereals should not be introduced until after the age of 9 months. At lunchtime babies should be fed with vegetables such as potato or carrot, or fruit such as apple. The vegetables can be fresh or frozen, and the fruit fresh or canned in natural juice. The vegetables should be boiled and the fruit stewed and then liquidized, mashed into purée or sieved. Feeding should start with half or one teaspoonful before or during the lunchtime feed and gradually increased.

When the infant has accepted these foods mothers should start to give a wider variety. Banana mashed with a fork is a favourite of many babies. Mashed hard-boiled eggs, soups and milk puddings should all be tried, with the emphasis on savoury

ABC of the First Year, Sixth edition. By B. Valman and R. Thomas. © 2009 Blackwell Publishing, ISBN: 978-1-4051-8037-5.

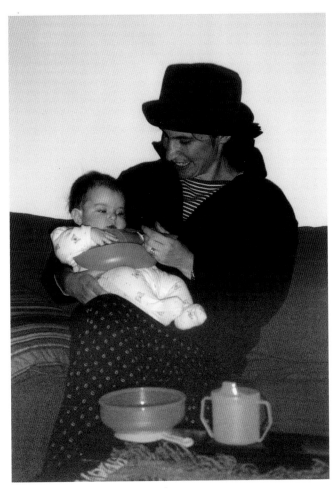

Figure 18.2 Feeding with a spoon while sitting on the mother's lap.

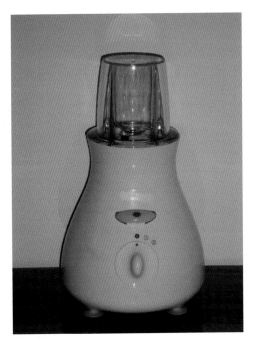

Figure 18.3 Electric liquidizer.

Box 18.1 **Menu at 6 months**

6–8 am	Milk
10 am	Milk *Baby cereal*
2 pm	Milk *Fruit or vegetable purée*
6 pm	Milk
10 pm	Milk

Box 18.2 **Menu at 7 to 8 months**

6 am	Milk feed
9–10 am	Cereal + milk *or* hard boiled egg
	Milk feed
1–2 pm	Minced/puréed meat or fish, puréed vegetables and potato, gravy
	Diluted fruit juice or milk feed
3–4 pm	Diluted fruit juice or water
5–6 pm	Fruit purée/mashed banana
	Custard or milk pudding
	Milk feed

---

flavours rather than sweet ones. Lightly boiled or scrambled eggs or omelettes should not be given, as there is a risk of salmonella infection.

Preparing food

Home-prepared foods are best. The mother knows what is in them and can prepare them easily and cheaply, as she can use a small portion of food cooked for the rest of the family. Sugar, salt and fat should not be added to the food being prepared for the baby. Many families have an electric liquidizer or food processor (Figure 18.3), but a manual blender is equally effective. A sieve is useful for making fruit and vegetable purées. If there is a deep freeze, time can be saved by preparing puréed food in bulk and storing individual portions for up to 3 months.

Cans, jars and packets of baby foods are useful but should not replace home-made foods. After opening, jars and cans should be kept in a refrigerator and used within 24 hours.

Iron deficiency is common during weaning but can be prevented by an appropriate diet. Iron from vegetables and cereals is not as well absorbed as that from meat. Sources of iron for vegetarians include breakfast cereals and other cereal products, pulses, green vegetables and nut purée.

7–8 months (Box 18.2)

At 7 months a greater variety of tastes and textures should be introduced. A little finely minced chicken, lamb, beef or liver may be given mixed with potato purée. Vegetables should be cooked until soft, then sieved, blended or liquidized until smooth. White fish can be boiled with milk and, after the bones have been removed, mashed in with potato or vegetable purée. Dahls such as chama dahl and dhudhi, lentils and rice can be given at this age, but should not include salt or hot spices (chilli, ginger and cloves), fat or oil.

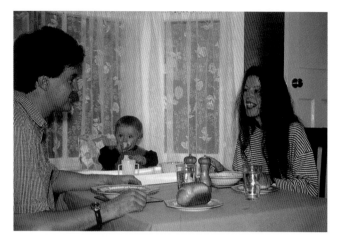

Figure 18.4 Sitting in highchair eating with the family.

Soup can be made with lentils, soft chick peas, carrots, cauliflower or potato, which can then be blended, liquidized or mashed. Grated cheese, cottage cheese, curd cheese or paneer may be given, mixed in with other foods, and mashed hard-boiled egg can be added to mashed potato. Babies often eat yoghurt plain, but they may need to be tempted with added fruit.

At around 8 months parents should start changing the texture of foods to encourage chewing. For example, meat and fish should be less finely minced and potatoes and other vegetables can be mashed rather than puréed. Babies should also be given hard foods such as a crust of bread, a piece of chapatti or pieces of apple, carrot and banana, which will encourage them to chew. These foods should always be given under supervision to make sure babies do not choke. Babies should not be given biscuits every day, as these may encourage the taste for sweet foods.

The timetable of feeds should also start to change at this age and the number of milk feeds should fall to a total intake of 450 mL of milk in 24 hours.

Babies often reject food. This may be because they are not used to a new taste or texture. However, it may also be because they are thirsty or because the food is too hot, or simply because they want to attract attention. Mothers should be told to keep trying with new foods and to give them in different ways. Babies who become constipated should be given more fruit and vegetables and water.

At about 8 months the baby can now sit in a highchair at the table with the rest of the family (Figure 18.4). Two-course meals at lunch and teatime should be introduced – for example, a savoury food followed by a fruit purée. The amount of milk will decrease as more solids are taken. Breastfeeding is continued, or infant formula milk should be given until the end of the first year. For food safety, see Box 18.3.

9–12 months

At this stage babies should be able to eat the same food as the rest of the family, though the food will have to be cut up or mashed. Food should not contain hot spices, particularly chilli, ginger or cloves, and not too much butter, ghee or oil. Each day the baby should have a pint of milk, or less if he or she eats some cheese or yoghurt; two

Box 18.3 **Food safety**

- Babies should never be left alone when eating, because of the risk of choking.
- Heated foods should be warm but not hot enough to burn a baby's mouth.
- It is not advisable to use a microwave oven to reheat food and drink. This is because 'hot spots' can occur in the middle of food if it is not thoroughly stirred after reheating.
- Eggs should be boiled until the white and yolk are solid (about 6 minutes).
- Peanuts and food containing peanuts or unrefined groundnut oil should not be given to infants from atopic families until they are at least 3 years of age or to infants who are atopic or allergic to peanuts.
- Whole nuts should not be given to children less than 4–5 years of age because of the risk of choking. However, smooth peanut butter or finely milled nuts are suitable.

small portions of meat, fish, poultry or eggs; some fruit, fresh fruit juice or vegetables; some cereals – for example, a cereal at breakfast and half a slice of bread at tea; and a small amount of butter or margarine. Babies should not be given too many sweet foods, particularly between meals, as they can cause overweight and tooth decay.

Vitamins

Babies who are breastfeeding after the age of 6 months and all infants receiving less than 1 pint (450 mL) of formula milk, which contains added vitamins, per day should receive supplementary drops of vitamins A, C and D until the age of 4 years.

Weaning and the prevention of obesity

The prevalence of obesity is increasing in both children and adults. Obese infants and children tend to become obese adults, who may suffer from diabetes, high blood pressure, heart disease and arthritis. Treatment to reduce established obesity in children is difficult and often unsuccessful. A planned approach to nutrition should be started at weaning and may be necessary throughout childhood to prevent obesity. This section will put the principles of healthy weaning foods into the context of nutrition during childhood.

Prevention

Milk has a bland taste because it has low concentrations of sugar, salt and fat. Weaning foods have a semi-solid or solid consistency but also have stronger flavours. The flavour of any food can be improved by adding sugar, salt or fat or all three. To make foods attractive and encourage children to eat a larger amount, food manufacturers add these substances to foods and mothers are tempted to follow this lead.

When a baby first receives weaning foods he or she is usually enthusiastic. As babies approach the age of 12 months their appetite falls and they may take a smaller amount or none of a

GIRLS BMI CHART

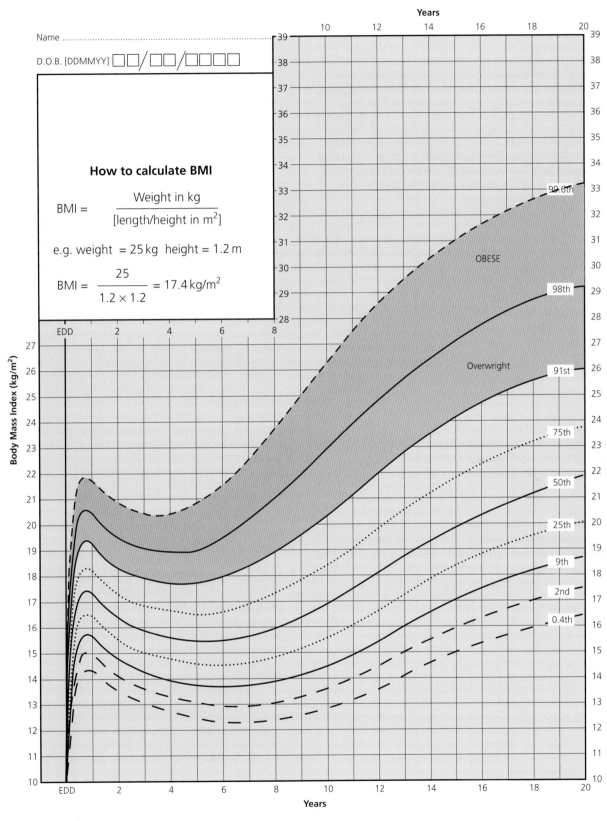

Figure 18.5 Girls BMI Chart.

particular food. The face, trunk and limbs become thinner due to a reduction in body fat. About this time infants enter the phase when they are trying to exert their individuality. The mother notices that the infant is becoming thinner as well as refusing food. The infant may be tempted with more tasty food in the mistaken idea that they need more food to continue to gain weight at the previous rate. These tempting foods often come from the mother's plate and may be high in sugar, salt and fat. The infant develops a taste for these highly flavoured foods and although they may eat only small quantities, they have developed a dislike for bland foods which will be lifelong and may lead to later obesity. A reduced appetite and becoming thinner at the age of a year is normal (Figure 18.5) and offering tempting food is not needed.

Early detection of obesity

If excessive weight gain is suspected, measure the child's height and weight, calculate body mass index (BMI) and plot it on a BMI chart (see Figure 18.5). If the BMI is above the 91st centile, refer the child to a paediatrician or dietician.

Management of obesity

Obesity is due to an excessive calorie intake with insufficient exercise. Some families have a strong history of obesity which may represent a genetic factor or a longstanding family custom to eat excessive calories. In less than 1% of children with obesity there is a causative disease, and this causes a reduction in height as well as obesity.

Reducing calorie intake

The goal is to reduce the child's weight or to maintain the present weight depending on the age and stage of growth. If the child is growing rapidly in height it may be necessary only to maintain the present weight as the growth in height will ensure that the weight gradually becomes appropriate for the increased height. The diet should be tailored to the child's preferences but avoiding hunger. The total energy intake should be reduced below the expenditure by reduction in fat and sugar. Snacks between meals should be avoided and food should not be offered as a reward for attaining a goal. In obese children a weight loss of 1 pound (450 g) per month

Table 18.1 Healthy diet for the whole family.

Base meals on starchy foods such as potatoes, bread, rice and pasta, choosing wholegrain where possible
Eat plenty of fibre-rich foods such as oats, beans, peas, lentils, grains, seeds, fruit and vegetables as well as wholegrain bread and brown rice and pasta
Eat at least five portions of a variety of fruit and vegetables a day in place of foods high in fat and calories (two portions for children under 2 years)
One portion of a protein food a day (fish, meat, eggs, cheese or other dairy food)
Choose low-fat foods
Avoid foods containing a lot of fat and sugar, such as fried food, sweetened drinks, sweets and chocolate. Some takeaways and fast foods contain a lot of fat and sugar
Eat regular meals as a family
Eat breakfast
Watch the portion sizes and how often food is eaten

can be achieved with the help of a dietician, but this is only helpful if it is sustainable. Self-monitoring and rewards for reaching goals are useful. Adoption of healthy eating by the whole family, especially if other members are overweight, is effective (see Table 18.1). Cooperation of the child and the whole family is essential.

Increasing exercise

A practical objective is to increase physical activity by at least 60 minutes each day, although not necessarily at one time. Sedentary behaviour such as watching television, using a computer or playing video games should be confined to 1 hour per day. The choice of physical activity should be agreed with the child and may involve informal exercise such as walking to school, cycling, or climbing stairs instead of using a lift. Regular structured activity may include sports at school, football, swimming or dancing. Activity of the whole family should be increased by walking to the local shops or park together.

Further reading

National Institute for Health and Clinical Excellence. (2006) *Obesity*. NICE clinical guideline 43. www.nice.org.uk/CG43

CHAPTER 19

Review at Six Weeks

OVERVIEW

- All infants are assessed within 48 hours of birth and at 6 weeks
- After asking specific questions on the infant's behaviour, the weight and head circumference are measured and plotted on the growth chart in the 'parent-held record'. Alertness, motor function, and the eyes, heart, hips and genitalia are examined
- Parental anxieties at other ages should be reviewed after reference to a developmental chart (page 90) and the infant referred to a secondary care specialist

The whole population is screened by examination in the neonatal period and at 6 weeks. Infants with an abnormality at these examinations and those at increased risk, for example born at extremely short gestation, are assessed later, especially at 8 months. A mother may suspect an abnormality at any age and Figure 19.5 below (page 90) can be used to determine whether the infant is within the normal range. At each visit for immunization the infant should be weighed and the weight plotted on a growth chart by a member of the health team who is able to interpret it. At the same visit the mother has an opportunity to express any anxieties about development and preventive healthcare advice can be given. Previously there were more fixed times for assessment of all infants but they have been replaced by reviews prompted by parents and health visitors. On average, an infant is seen by the family doctor nine times in the first year and each visit provides an opportunity for a review. When the infant is 4 months, the health visitor produces a plan for times of assessment depending on the vulnerability of the infant, for example postnatal depression.

Early detection of an abnormality may provide an opportunity for early treatment, for example physiotherapy for cerebral palsy, and for the provision of educational and social help. It allows genetic counselling for the family, including future pregnancies.

Developmental examinations should be considered on two levels: the surveillance of an apparently healthy population; and the detailed assessment of infants referred from primary examinations because of suspected abnormalities. Primary examinations, which

should cover all infants in the district, are best performed by the family doctor. In some districts specially trained health visitors do this work, especially for infants whose parents will not visit the surgery or clinic. Some clinics are run jointly by a family doctor and health visitor, who often has wide experience of managing feeding and behaviour problems.

Infants found to be abnormal at the primary examination need to be referred to a doctor with a special interest in developmental assessment. This may be the community or the hospital paediatrician. The more detailed examination performed at this stage may need a team of paramedical staff.

A mother who considers that her infant has an abnormality of hearing, sight or development must be sent straight to the specialist, because she cannot be reassured until a detailed assessment has been performed, which usually needs several members of the team. The mother is likely to be right.

Primary examination

Infants in the normal population should be assessed within 48 hours of birth and at 6 weeks. Preterm infants should be examined about 6 weeks after the expected date of delivery, when their development should be the same as that of a 6 week infant born at term. The primary examination should take no more than about 15 minutes and should be confined to items that have prognostic significance.

A health visitor visits the family at home, usually when the baby is between 10 and 14 days old. Health visitors are trained nurses who have specialist qualifications in child and family health. They are part of the primary care team which includes the family doctor and practice nurse. The health visitor gives the mother a 'parent-held' manual record that, if completed correctly by professionals and parents, is a complete record of a child's health. All child health surveillance data, the dates of immunizations, outcomes of visits to general practitioners and hospitals, and contacts with other healthcare professionals can be recorded. Some health advice is also included throughout this record. In addition, the Department of Health's book *Birth to Five Years*, which is given to all first-time mothers, is an excellent manual on child health for all parents (and junior doctors).

The 6-week examination should include a physical examination and assessment of alertness, vision and motor function. The checks

ABC of the First Year, Sixth edition. By B. Valman and R. Thomas. © 2009 Blackwell Publishing, ISBN: 978-1-4051-8037-5.

6–8 weeks review

Review at 6–8 weeks
For parent to complete:

This review is done by your health visitor and/or a doctor. Below is a list of things you may want to discuss when you see them. However, if you are worried about your child's health, growth or development you can contact your health visitor or doctor at any time.

Health topics for discussion	Immunisation ☐
	Recognition of illness ☐
	Nutrition ☐
	Activities to aid development ☐
	Dangers: fire, scalds, falls, overheating ☐
Tick ☑	Good child rearing practices ☐

Circle 'yes' or 'no' or 'not sure'

Do you feel well yourself?	Yes/no/not sure
Do you have any worries about **feeding** your baby?	Yes/no/not sure
Do you have any concerns about your baby's **weight** gain?	Yes/no/not sure
Does your baby watch your face and follow with his/her eyes?	Yes/no/not sure
Does your baby turn towards the light?	Yes/no/not sure
Does your baby smile at you?	Yes/no/not sure
Do you think your baby can hear you?	Yes/no/not sure
Is your baby started by loud noises?	Yes/no/not sure
Are there any problems in looking after your baby?	Yes/no/not sure
Do you have any other worries about your baby?	Yes/no/not sure

Comment _____

How are you feeding your baby?   Breast/bottle/mixed

**Keep hot drinks away from children
Use a coiled-flex kettle.**

**Check the water before you bath your baby.
Hot water can scald your baby badly.**

Review at 6–8 weeks
*Please place a sticker (if available) otherwise write in space provided.

Surname
First names
NHS number   Local no
Address   Sex   M/F
_____ Postcode _____ D.O.B. _/_/_
G.P.   Code
H.V.   Code

Any previous ongoing medical problems? NO ☐   Yes ☐
If 'Yes' please specify (1) _____ (2) _____ (3) _____
ICD Code

Date of examination _____ /_____ /_____
Age in weeks _____
Name of examiner

Examiner code number   Examination centre

WEIGHT _____ kg _____ centile
HEAD CIRC. _____ cm _____ centile
FEEDING _____ Breast/Bottle/Mixed

ITEM	GUIDE TO CONTENT	CODE (Ring one)*	COMMENT
Response	Alertness	S P O T R N	
Vision	Eyes, Follows. Red reflex.	S P O T R N	
Hearing	Ears, Risk factor, Parents observations	S P O T R N	
Motor	Prone posture	S P O T R N	
Speech/Lang.	Vocalisation	S P O T R N	
Behaviour	Social smile, Cry, Sleep	S P O T R N	
Hips		S P O T R N	
Genitalia	Testicular descent	S P O T R N	
Heart	Heart murmurs, Femoral pulses	S P O T R N	

*(If one or more codes seem to apply select the last one, e.g. R takes priority over T, T over O etc.)
S = Satisfactory *(normal result)*
P = Problem *(significant condition on record)*
O = Observation *(special recall arranged)*
T = Treatment or investigation underway
R = Referred to any community or hospital service
N = Not examined for this item

Referred to   (1)_____ (2)_____
               (3)_____
Special recall in _____   _____

6–8 weeks

White copy: Stay in Record   Yellow copy: to Child Health Office
Pink copy: to GP/HV

Figure 19.1 Review at 6–8 weeks.

should be carried out as part of clinical care and not be regarded as 'pass or fail' examinations. A simple form is useful for recording the information quickly (Figure 19.1).

Of greatest importance is the child's alertness, interest in their surroundings, responsiveness and ability to concentrate. The physical examination of the infant should always include measurement of weight and head circumference. These values, plotted on a growth chart, will show at a glance whether the infant's growth is normal.

Weighing and measuring

Being undressed and weighed is often the most worrying part of the visit to the child. Weighing the child in vest and napkin reduces upset and time taken. Weights of the vest and napkin (Box 19.1) should be subtracted from the total weight. Suitable scales that are checked regularly are an essential piece of equipment.

In very young infants it is easier to measure head circumference than length. The measurement should be made, using a paper tape measure, around the occipitofrontal circumference (the largest circumference). Measurements can then be plotted on a growth chart together with weights.

The length of infants aged under 2 years is measured on a special measuring board and accurate results can be obtained only when there are two dedicated measurers present. One has to hold the infant's head against the top board while the other brings the foot-board up to the child's feet while stretching him or her out. When the child is old enough to stand a special stadiometer can be used to measure height, but careful attention to detail is necessary for reproducible results.

Vision and squint

The infant's visual attention is engaged by the examiner crouching about 60 cm in front of the infant so that their eyes are on the same level. When the examiner slowly moves his or her head a short distance to one side then the other, the normal infant will continue to hold their gaze (Figure 19.2). Failure to do so is abnormal but may be due to something distracting the infant. Infants who fail to follow must be examined again 2 weeks later. Possible causes include lack of stimulation at home, delay in development or blindness.

The second routine test at this age is the detection of the red reflex. If a bright ophthalmoscope is held about 45 cm away from an infant's eye, with the observer looking down the beam of light, a bright red reflex is normally seen in a fair-skinned infant and a

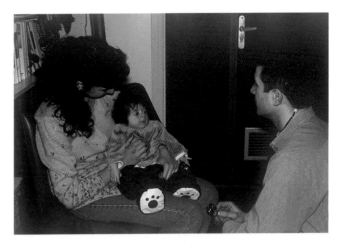

Figure 19.2 Infant following movements of the examiner.

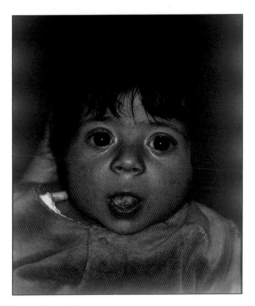

Figure 19.3 Looking at the camera.

dark red or grey reflex in an infant with a dark skin. Absence of the reflex indicates an abnormality of the refractive media and requires urgent referral to an ophthalmologist. An infant who does not fixate on the examiner's face at the second visit should be referred to a developmental specialist (Figure 19.3).

In a young infant a squint can be noticed by observing the position of the light reflex on each cornea when a torch is shone into the eyes. Normally the reflex should be in the centre of each pupil or at a corresponding point on each cornea. If there is a possibility of a squint, movements of the eyes should be assessed and the cornea, lens and fundi should be examined. An infant with a squint needs to be referred to an ophthalmologist.

Motor function

The baby should be placed prone on a couch; normally they will lift their head for a few seconds, though some infants may take

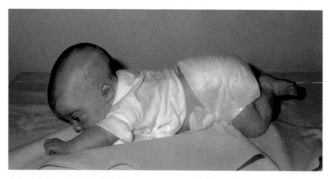

Figure 19.4 Lifting the head.

a few minutes to do so (Figure 19.4). Infants who usually sleep prone are more advanced in lifting their heads than others. If the infant does not eventually their head they need to be re-examined 2 weeks later.

When the infant is held in the prone position, the head rises to the same plane as the trunk and the legs do not fall vertically.

Other assessments

The testes and hips should be examined by the methods described for the newborn infant. It is difficult to detect an abnormal hip

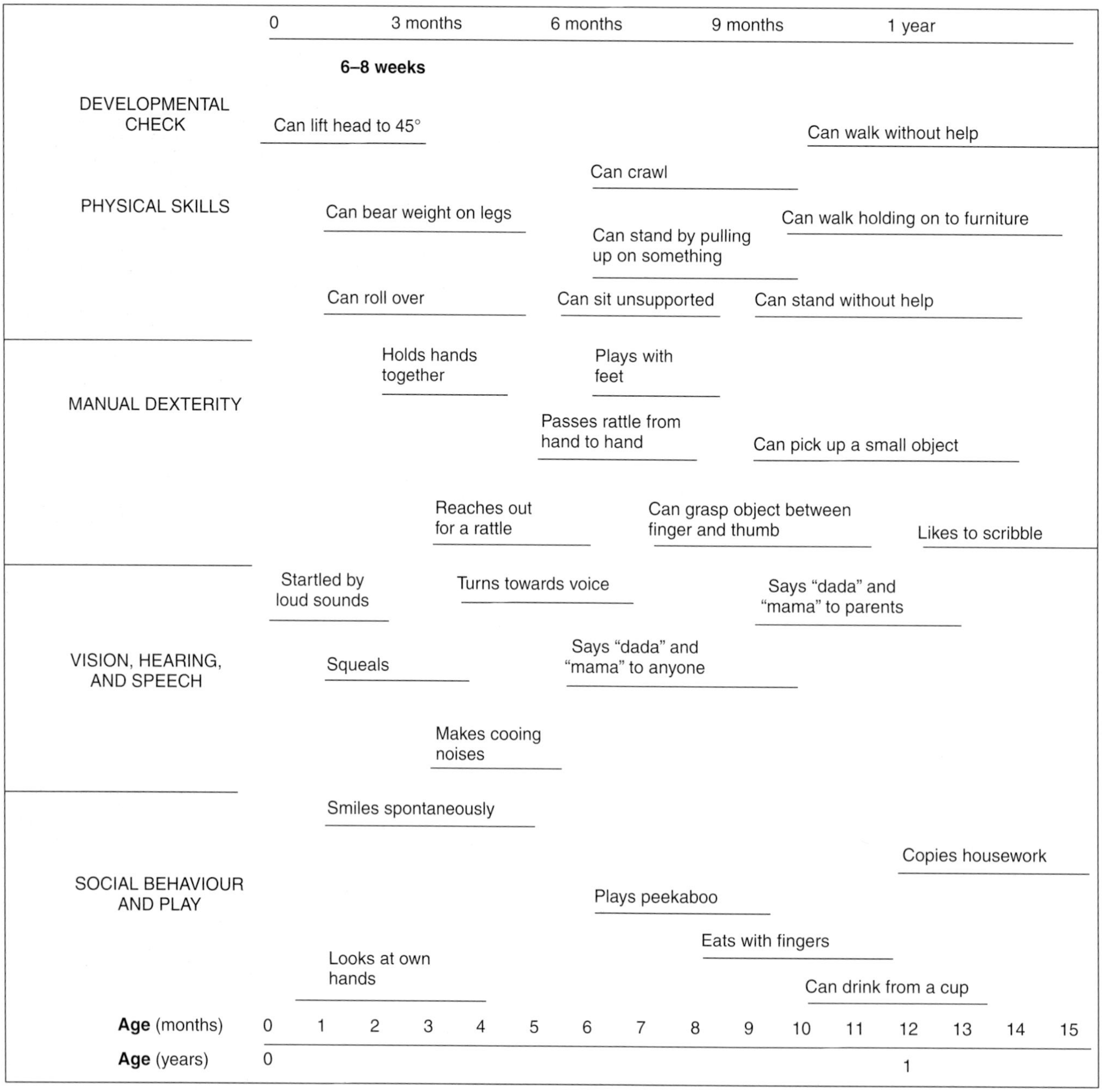

	0	3 months	6 months	9 months	1 year
		6–8 weeks			
DEVELOPMENTAL CHECK		Can lift head to 45°			Can walk without help
PHYSICAL SKILLS		Can bear weight on legs	Can crawl	Can stand by pulling up on something	Can walk holding on to furniture
		Can roll over	Can sit unsupported	Can stand without help	
MANUAL DEXTERITY		Holds hands together	Plays with feet		
			Passes rattle from hand to hand	Can pick up a small object	
		Reaches out for a rattle		Can grasp object between finger and thumb	Likes to scribble
VISION, HEARING, AND SPEECH	Startled by loud sounds	Turns towards voice		Says "dada" and "mama" to parents	
		Squeals	Says "dada" and "mama" to anyone		
			Makes cooing noises		
SOCIAL BEHAVIOUR AND PLAY		Smiles spontaneously			Copies housework
			Plays peekaboo		
		Looks at own hands		Eats with fingers	
				Can drink from a cup	
Age (months)	0 1 2 3 4	5 6 7 8	9 10 11	12 13	14 15
Age (years)	0			1	

Figure 19.5 Range of ages for attainment of milestones.

at the age of 6 weeks and ideally the condition should have been detected in the newborn infant.

Cardiac murmurs should be sought for and the femoral pulses checked. The normal infant will respond to sounds by stopping crying, opening his or her eyes widely or by a startle reflex, depending on the intensity of the sound.

Patterns of development in childhood

Progress in a particular field does not occur gradually but in spurts, and when one skill is advancing quickly others tend to go into abeyance.

There is considerable variation in the range of normal development, but among the children who fall outside the normal range there are some who later turn out to be normal (Figure 19.5). The children who fall into this group need examining more closely and more often to determine which are definitely abnormal. They should be referred to developmental specialists.

Lack of appropriate stimulation may cause delay in physical, intellectual, or social development. This factor must be taken into account if the mother has a learning disability or has had puerperal depression. These children advance rapidly when the mother is given advice on handling them or they are placed in a better environment. Delayed speech development, probably the commonest disability of childhood, may be prevented by encouraging parents to talk to their infants from birth.

No child has impaired intelligence if development is delayed in a single field and normal in all others. A child who is slow at learning will be delayed in all fields, except sometimes in walking. Intelligence cannot be assessed accurately until the age of about 4½ years and before that age it is best to use the term developmental delay.

Children vary in the ages when they acquire physical, mental and social skills. Figure 19.5 shows the normal ranges. Although abilities usually appear in a specific order, in some families one aspect of development may be unusually early or late. In these children, sitting, walking or speech may be late but development in all other fields is normal. Finding that an infant is not sitting by a certain age does not necessarily mean that he or she is abnormal, as they may show a variation of normal development. These children fall into a group who are late in reaching a developmental milestone and it is reasonable that they should be referred for a further assessment to exclude more sinister problems.

If parents suspect that a child may have delay in an aspect of development, the chart can be used to determine whether all or some abilities fall within the normal range. The child's age is marked at the foot of the chart and by placing a vertical line from that age the child's abilities can be compared with the normal range. Occasionally a stage is missed out and the child may walk without having crawled.

Equipment for examining children

Most of the equipment needed for examining and assessing children is cheap, but its use would greatly improve the quality of care: scales, disposable paper tape measures, measuring rod, torch,

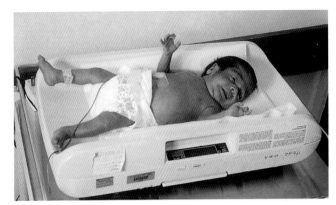

(a)

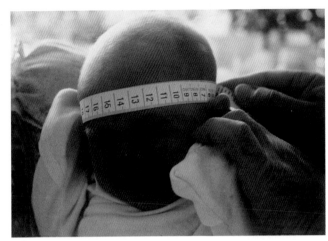

(b)

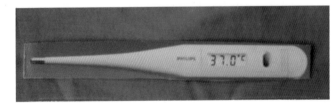

(c)

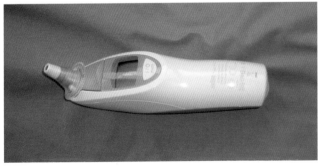

(d)

Figure 19.6 Essential equipment: (a) scales; (b) disposable paper tape; (c) digital thermometer; (d) aural thermometer; (e) building blocks; (f) books; (g) ophthalmoscope; (h) picture on ceiling; (i) auriscope.

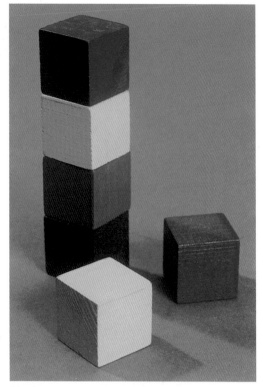

(e)

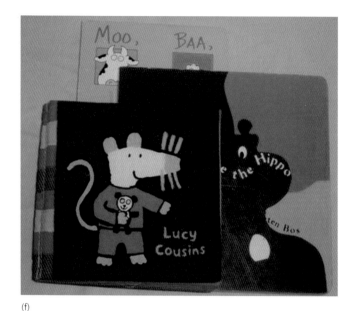

(f)

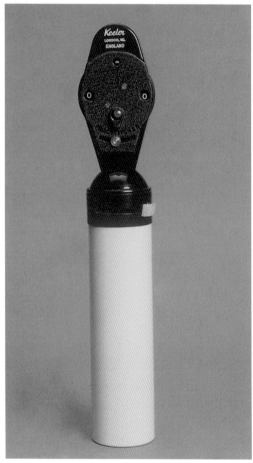

(g)

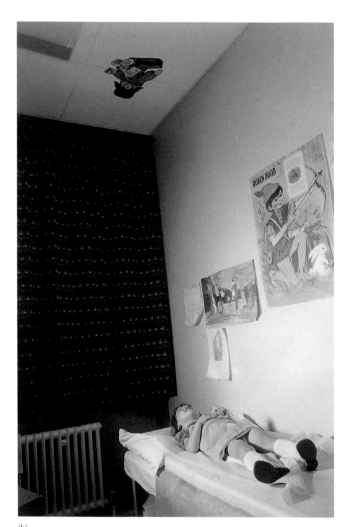

(h)

Figure 19.6 Continued.

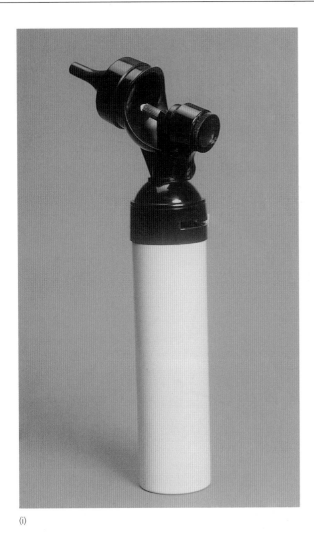

(i)

Figure 19.6 (continued) Auriscope.

auriscope, spatulas, centile charts, 1 inch cubes, books, miniature cups and saucers, small table and chair, pictures on the ceiling, toys (including wooden puzzles, pencils and paper), heel prick equipment and ophthalmoscope (Figure 19.6).

Further reading

Blair M, Isaacs A. (2003) Evidence-based child health surveillance for the National Child Health Promotion Programme. *Current Paediatrics* 13 issue 4.

Hall DMB, Elliman D. (2006) *Health For all Children*, revised 4th edn. Oxford University Press, Oxford. www.health-for-all-children.co.uk

Review at Eight Months

Mothers are asked whether they have any problems and whether the infants have had any illnesses since the last examination (Figure 20.1). They are also asked whether the infants are making sounds and the details of their diet, in particular whether they are chewing solids.

As at 6 weeks, the infant's alertness and interest are checked. Head circumference and weight should be measured and plotted on the growth chart.

Vision

Eye movements should be noted. If a squint is suspected, the position of the light reflex in each cornea should be observed; if there is a squint, the reflex will be in a different position in each eye. While the infant looks at an object one eye is covered with the doctor's hand. If the eye that is not being covered moves to fixate the object, that eye has an overt squint. The covering hand is slowly removed and if that eye moves to fixate the object, there is a latent squint. If a squint is seen or suspected at any time the infant should be seen by an ophthalmologist.

Near vision may be tested by placing a raisin or pellet of paper about 20 cm in front of an infant and watching whether he or she reaches out to grab it (Figure 20.2). Testing distant vision

is time-consuming at this age and is usually performed only at specialist clinics.

Motor development

From the prone position infants should get up on their wrists (Figure 20.3). When pulled from the supine position they should be able to sit spontaneously for a minute or two. Normal children can sit without help by the age of 8 months. Infants should also be able to take their weight on their legs when they are held standing (Figure 20.4).

If a cube is placed in front of the infant he should grab it with his whole hand. This test should be tried for both the right and the left hand, and the infant should transfer the object from one hand to the other. Infants who perform all these tests normally but are not sitting spontaneously should be seen again 2 months later.

A dislocated hip will show reduction of abduction and a proximal displacement of the lower buttock crease. Bilateral dislocation is hard to detect clinically but radiographs of the hips will confirm the diagnosis at this age.

Hearing

All infants are screened in the neonatal period by the otoacustic emissions (OAE) test. In addition high-risk infants, including preterm infants, have an auditory brainstem response (ABR) test at that stage. If there is an increased risk of deafness (Table 20.1), another hearing test is performed at 8 months. A suspicion of poor hearing or delayed development of speech or other skills are indications for a hearing test appropriate to the child's age (Table 20.2).

Pattern of development

Most normal children sit unaided by the age of 8 months. African children tend to advance in most aspects of motor development faster than other children up to the age of about 7 months. In some families one aspect of development – for example, sitting, walking or speech – may be unusually early or late, the development in all other fields being normal.

ABC of the First Year, Sixth edition. By B. Valman and R. Thomas. © 2009 Blackwell Publishing, ISBN: 978-1-4051-8037-5.

Review at 8–9 months
For parent to complete:

8–9 months review

This review is done by your health visitor and/or a doctor. Below is a list of things you may want to discuss when you see them. However, if you are worried about your child's health, growth or development you can contact your health visitor or doctor at any time.

Health topics for discussion:

Tick ☑

Accident prevention: choking, scalds, safety in cars and house, sunburn
Dental advice
Developmental needs
Nutrition, etc.

Circle 'yes' or 'no' or 'not sure'

Do you feel well yourself?	Yes/no/not sure
Do you have any worries about your child's health?	Yes/no/not sure
Do you have any worries about how your baby is feeding?	Yes/no/not sure
Are you happy your baby is gaining weight?	Yes/no/not sure
Do you have any worries about your baby's development?	Yes/no/not sure
Is your baby sitting alone?	Yes/no/not sure
Is your baby using both hands?	Yes/no/not sure
Does your baby babble (Ba-ba, de-de, etc.)?	Yes/no/not sure
Have you any worries about your baby's eyesight?	Yes/no/not sure
Can s/he recognise carer at a distance?	Yes/no/not sure
Have you noticed a squint (eyes not moving together?)	
Do you think your baby can hear you?	
Comment _____	

Are all your child's immunisations up to date?   Yes/no

Do you have fire guards to stop your child touching heaters and open fires?

Review at 8–9 months

*Please place a sticker (if available) otherwise write in space provided.

Surname
First names
NHS number   Local no
Address   Sex   M/F
                     Postcode   D.O.B. _/_/_
G.P.   Code
H.V.   Code

Date of examination _____ /_____ /_____
Age in weeks _____
Name of examiner

Examiner code number   Examination centre

WEIGHT _____ kg _____ centile
HEAD CIRC. _____ cm _____ centile

Any previous ongoing medical problems? NO ☐   Yes ☐
If 'Yes' please specify (1) _____ (2) _____ (3) _____
ICD Code

ITEM	GUIDE TO CONTENT	CODE (Ring one)*	COMMENT
Physical	Parents observations. Diet.	S P O T R N	
Vision	Eye movements. Visual behaviour. Cover test.	S P O T R N	
Hearing	Appropriate test.	S P O T R N	
Locomotion	Sitting. Some weight bearing.	S P O T R N	
Manipulation	Transfers. Uses both hands.	S P O T R N	
Speech/Lang.	Babble. Responds to speech.	S P O T R N	
Behaviour	Knows strangers. Enjoys mirror image Socialisation. Alertness	S P O T R N	
Hips	Check for CDH	S P O T R N	
Genitalia	Testicular descent (Ring 'N' for girl)	S P O T R N	

*(If one or more codes seem to apply select the last one, e.g. R takes priority over T, T over O etc.)

S = Satisfactory *(normal result)*
P = Problem *(significant condition on record)*
O = Observation *(special recall arranged)*
T = Treatment or investigation underway
R = Referred to any community or hospital service
N = Not examined for this item

Referred to   (1)_____ (2)_____
              (3)_____
Special recall in _____ wks/mths   Signature _____

White copy: Stay in Record   Yellow copy: to Child Health Office
Pink copy: to GP/HV

8–9 months

Figure 20.1 Review at 8–9 months.

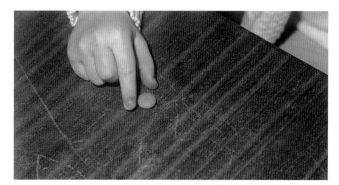

Figure 20.2 Near vision being tested.

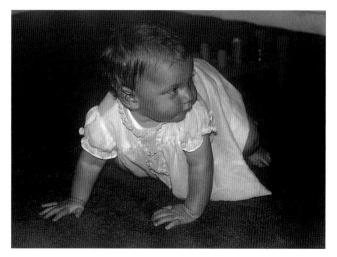

Figure 20.3 Resting on the wrists in the prone position.

Table 20.1 Risk factors for hearing loss.

Neonatal
Family history of hereditary childhood sensorineural hearing loss
In-utero infections (toxoplasmosis, rubella, cytomegalovirus, herpes simplex, syphilis)
Craniofacial anomalies and syndromes associated with hearing loss
Birthweight less than 1500 g
Hyperbilirubinaemia requiring exchange transfusion
Congenital hypothyroidism
Ototoxic medications (aminoglycosides)
Bacterial meningitis or encephalitis
Postnatal asphyxia (APGAR less than 5 at 1 minute or 6 at 5 minutes)
Mechanical ventilation lasting 5 days or more

Later additional factors
Recurrent otitis media
Measles, influenza, chickenpox, mumps
Head injury
Noise exposure

Finding that an infant is not sitting by a certain age does not necessarily mean that he or she is abnormal, as this may be a variation of normal development. These children fall into a group who are late in reaching a developmental milestone and it is reasonable that they should be referred for further examination to exclude more sinister problems.

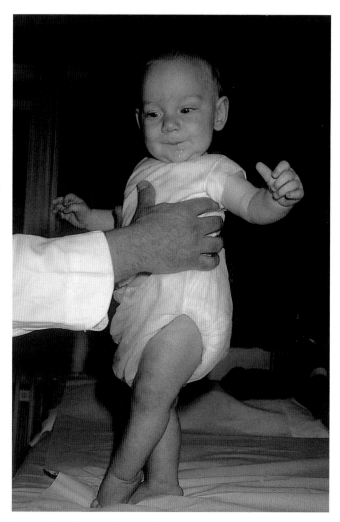

Figure 20.4 Taking weight on the feet.

Table 20.2 Appropriate hearing tests for age.

Test	Age	Procedure
Otoacustic emissions	Any age	Sounds transmitted from generator to inner ear by device in ear. Echo is recorded
Auditory brainstem response	Any age	Device in ear makes sounds and the response of the 8th nerve is recorded from scalp electrodes
Distraction	6–18 months	Infant turns head to various noise stimuli
Visual reinforcement audiometry	6–32 months	Sounds presented through earphones or speakers and child is trained to turn to sound with a reward
Tympanometry (part of evaluation but not strictly a hearing test)	Any age	Tests mobility of drum and detects middle ear disease

Further reading

McCormick B. (2004) *Paediatric Audiology*, 3rd edn. WHURR Publishers, London.

CHAPTER 21

Respiratory Infections in the Older Infant

Infection of the respiratory tract is a common cause of illness of infants. Although pathogens are often not confined to anatomical boundaries, the infections may be classified as: (a) upper respiratory tract – common cold, tonsillitis, and otitis media (Figure 21.1); (b) middle respiratory tract – acute laryngitis and epiglottitis; and (c) lower respiratory tract – bronchitis, bronchiolitis and pneumonia.

Upper respiratory tract infection is usually the least serious condition but blockage of the nose by mucus may completely obstruct the airway in those infants who cannot breathe through their mouths. Middle respiratory tract infection may totally obstruct airflow at the narrowest part of the airway. Lower respiratory tract infection produces trivial signs initially but may be lethal within a few hours.

Viruses, which cause most respiratory tract infections, and bacterial infections produce similar clinical illness. Different viruses may produce an identical clinical picture or the same virus may cause different clinical syndromes. Clinically it may not be possible to determine whether the infection is due to viruses, bacteria, or both. If the infection is suspected of being bacterial, it is safest to prescribe an antibiotic, as the results of virus studies are often received after the acute symptoms have passed. The commonest bacterial pathogens are pneumococci, *Haemophilus influenzae*, group A β-haemolytic streptococci, and *Staphylococcus aureus*. Group B streptococci, Gram-negative bacteria and anaerobic bacteria are less common.

ABC of the First Year, Sixth edition. By B. Valman and R. Thomas. © 2009 Blackwell Publishing, ISBN: 978-1-4051-8037-5.

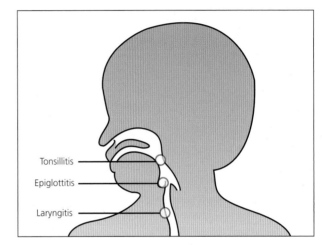

Figure 21.1 Sites of infection in the upper respiratory tract.

Box 21.1 **Main symptoms of common cold**

- Sneezing
- Nasal discharge
- Cough
- Fever (rare)

Common cold (coryza)

Preschool children have at least 3–6 colds each year. The main symptoms are sneezing, nasal discharge, cough and, rarely, fever (Box 21.1). Nasal obstruction in infants who cannot breathe through their mouths may cause feeding difficulties and, rarely, brief periods of apnoea. Similar symptoms may occur in the early phases of infection with rotavirus and be followed by vomiting and diarrhoea. Postnasal discharge may produce coughing. The commonest complication is acute otitis media, but secondary bacterial infection of the lower respiratory tract sometimes occurs.

There is no specific treatment for the common cold and antibiotics should be avoided. If an infant is not able to feed due to nasal obstruction from mucus, two drops of 0.9% sodium chloride solution can be instilled into each nostril before feeds three times daily. This will wash the mucus into the back of the pharynx and relieve the obstruction. There is a danger with nasal drops that they will run down into the lower respiratory tract and carry the infection there.

Tonsillitis and pharyngitis

In children aged under 3 years the commonest presenting features of tonsillitis are fever and refusal to eat, but a febrile convulsion may occur at the onset. Older children may complain of a sore throat or enlarged cervical lymph nodes, which may or may not be painful. Viral and bacterial causes cannot be distinguished clinically as a purulent follicular exudate may be present in both. Ideally, a throat swab should be sent to the laboratory before starting treatment, to determine a bacterial cause for the symptoms and to help to indicate the pathogens currently in the community. There has been a recurrence of group A haemolytic streptococci in outbreaks of sore throat and a more liberal use of penicillin is justified. As this organism is the only important bacterium causing tonsillitis, penicillin is the drug of choice and the only justification for using another antibiotic is a convincing history of hypersensitivity to penicillin. In that case the alternative is erythromycin. In the absence of an outbreak of group A streptococcus infection the indication for oral penicillin is fever or severe systemic symptoms. The drug should be continued for at least 10 days if a streptococcal infection is confirmed (Figure 21.2). Parents often stop the drug after a few days as the symptoms have often abated and the medicine is unpalatable. The organism is not eradicated unless a full 10-day course is given.

Viral infections often produce two peaks on the temperature chart (Figure 21.3).

An extensive thick white shaggy exudate on the tonsils (sometimes invading the pharynx) suggests infectious mononucleosis and a full blood count, examination of the blood film, and a Monospot test are indicated. Although rare in UK, a membranous exudate on the tonsils suggests diphtheria and an urgent expert opinion should be sought.

Paracetamol given every 6 hours during the first 24–48 hours reduces fever and discomfort. If it is not effective, it can be replaced by ibuprofen. While there is dysphagia the child may prefer to take only fluids, but ice cream, yogurt or jelly may be accepted.

A peritonsillar abscess (quinsy) is now extremely rare. It displaces the tonsil medially so that the swollen soft palate obscures the tonsil and the uvula is displaced across the midline. The advice of an otolaryngology surgeon is needed urgently.

Otitis media

Pain is the main symptom of acute otitis media and is one of the few causes of a fretful infant who cries all night. The pain is relieved if the drum ruptures. Viruses probably cause over half the cases of acute otitis, but a viral or bacterial origin cannot be distinguished clinically. The commonest bacteria are pneumococci, group A β-haemolytic streptococci and *H. influenzae.*

Children are often fascinated by the light of the auriscope and the auriscope speculum can be placed on a doll or the child's forearm for reassurance (Figure 21.4). Gentleness is essential and the speculum should never be pushed too far into the external meatus because this causes pain. If the pinna is pulled gently outwards and downwards to open the meatal canal, the tympanic membrane is visible with the tip of the speculum in the outer end of the meatus. In early cases of otitis media there are dilated vessels over the upper and posterior part of the drum (Figure 21.5). Later, the tympanic membrane becomes red, congested and bulging, and the light reflex is lost. Swelling or tenderness behind the pinna should always be sought, as mastoiditis can be easily missed.

Amoxycillin is the first choice of antibiotic but erythromycin is given if the child is sensitive to one of the penicillins. If there is no improvement in the symptoms or appearance of the drums after 2 or 3 days, another antibiotic should be substituted. Amoxycillin with clavulanic acid or cefalexin are the second-line drugs. The duration of the course of antibiotics is controversial. The most common view is that antibiotics should be given for 5 days and the ears examined again before the course is stopped. There is some evidence that short courses of 3–5 days of antibiotics given at high doses may be as effective as the longer courses. Ideally, a hearing test should be performed 3 months after each

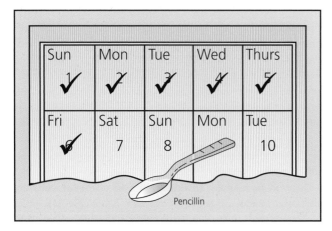

Figure 21.2 Antibiotics should be taken regularly.

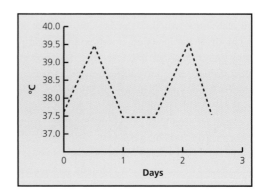

Figure 21.3 Temperature chart in a viral infection.

attack of acute otitis media to detect residual deafness and 'glue ear'. One study showed that after the first attack of acute otitis media in infants, which was treated with antimicrobial agents, 40% of patients had no middle ear effusion after 1 month and 90% after 3 months.

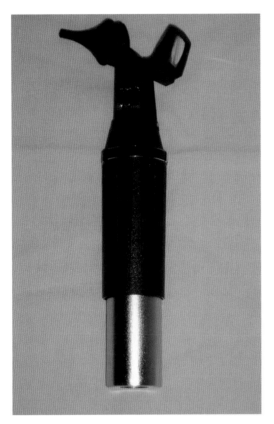

Figure 21.4 Auriscope.

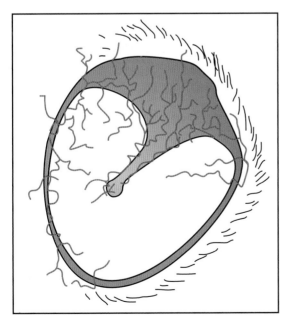

Figure 21.5 Acute otitis media.

Stridor

Stridor is noisy breathing caused by obstruction in the pharynx, larynx or trachea. It may be distinguished from partial obstruction of the bronchi by the absence of rhonchi. Although most cases are due to acute laryngitis and may resolve with the minimum of care, similar features may be due to a foreign body and may cause sudden death.

Stridor is recognized as one of the most ominous signs in childhood. Any doctor should be able to recognise the sound over the telephone and arrange to see the child immediately. Examination of the throat may precipitate total obstruction of the airway and should be attempted only in the presence of an anaesthetist and facilities for intubation.

A glance at the child will show whether urgent treatment is needed or whether there is time for a detailed history to be taken. The doctor needs to know when the symptoms started and whether there is nasal discharge or cough. Choking over food, especially peanuts, or the abrupt onset of symptoms after playing alone with small objects suggests that a foreign body is present.

During the taking of the history and the examination mothers should remain near their children and be encouraged to hold them and to talk to them. All unpleasant procedures, such as venepuncture, should be avoided (Box 21.2). This reduces the possibility of struggling, which may precipitate complete airway obstruction. Agitation and struggling raise the peak flow rate and move secretions, which results in increased hypoxia and the production of more secretions.

Acute laryngotracheitis

Acute laryngitis causes partial obstruction of the larynx. It is characterized by inspiratory and expiratory stridor (noisy breathing), cough and hoarseness. The laryngeal obstruction is due to oedema, spasm and secretions. Affected children are usually aged 6 months to 3 years, and the symptoms are most severe in the early hours of the morning. Recession of the intercostal spaces indicates significant obstruction and cyanosis or drowsiness shows that total obstruction of the airway is imminent.

A child often improves considerably after inhaling steam, which is provided easily by turning on the hot taps in the bathroom. Mild cases may be treated successfully at home using this method, but children must be visited every few hours to determine whether they are deteriorating and need to be admitted to hospital. Continuous stridor or recession demands urgent hospital admission (Figure 21.6). Hypoxaemia or thirst may cause restlessness and should be corrected and sedatives avoided (Box 21.3). Infants with moderate or severe symptoms should be given a single oral dose of dexamethasone or prednisolone before transfer to hospital. In hospital dexamethasone is given orally or by injection or budesonide

Box 21.2 **Procedures to be avoided in the presence of stridor**

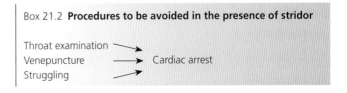

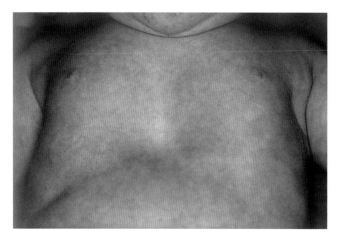

Figure 21.6 Substernal recession.

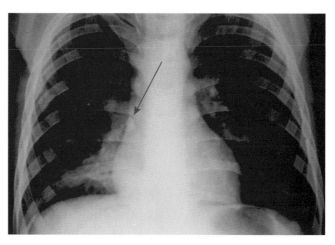

Figure 21.8 Foreign body in right main bronchus (tooth).

Box 21.3 **Restlessness could indicate:**

- hypoxia
- thirst
- hunger
- fear

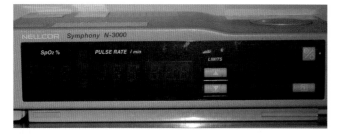

Figure 21.7 Oximeter for measuring blood oxygen saturation.

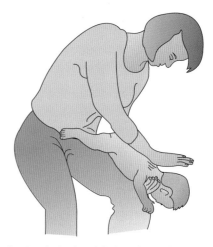

Figure 21.9 Slapping the back to dislodge a foreign body.

by nebulization. If the symptoms are severe or the infant deteriorates despite the steroid treatment, nebulized adrenaline is given and repeated after 30 minutes if necessary. Monitoring in a high-dependency unit or intensive care unit is needed to detect a possible recurrence of the obstruction (Figure 21.7). Rarely, the obstruction needs to be relieved by passing an endotracheal tube or performing a tracheostomy.

Acute laryngotracheitis is usually caused by a viral infection and therefore infants with mild symptoms do not need antibiotics. In a few cases *Staph. aureus* or *H. influenzae* is present and the associated septicaemia makes the child appear very ill. Bacterial infection is characterized by plaques of debris and pus on the surface of the trachea, partially obstructing it, just below the vocal cords. Acute epiglottitis and acute laryngitis may be indistinguishable clinically since stridor and progressive upper airway obstruction are the main features of both. If bacterial infection is suspected cefotaxime is given intravenously. Some paediatricians give steroids and an antibiotic.

Children with epiglottitis are usually aged over 2 years; drooling and dysphagia are common, and the child usually wants to sit upright. When the obstruction is very severe, the stridor becomes ominously quieter. There is usually an associated septicaemia with *H. influenzae*. Epiglottitis is now rare due to the Hib vaccine.

Other causes of stridor

Even if the symptoms have settled and there are no abnormal signs, a history of the onset of sudden choking or coughing can never be ignored. A radiograph of the neck and chest should be taken and may show a hypertranslucent lung obstructed by a foreign body, a shift of the mediastinum or, less commonly, collapse of part of the lung or a radio-opaque foreign body (Figure 21.8). The radiograph may be considered normal. Bronchoscopy may be needed to exclude a foreign body even if the chest radiograph appears to be normal. Stridor in a child who has had scalds or burns or has inhaled steam from a kettle suggests that intubation or tracheostomy may be needed urgently.

If the cause of stridor is likely to be a foreign body, the object should be removed immediately by an ENT surgeon and anaesthetist in the main or accident and emergency operating theatre. No attempt should be made to look at the mouth or throat or remove the object, as the struggling that may follow may impact the object and prove fatal. A first aid measure usually performed before arrival is to slap the infant's back between the shoulder blades while holding the infant upside down by the legs (Figure 21.9). The child should remain in the position he or she finds most comfortable, which is usually upright. Forceful attempts to make the child lie flat – for example, for a radiograph – may result in complete airway obstruction.

Infants with congenital laryngeal stridor, which is due to loose aryepiglottic folds, usually have inspiratory stridor only. The symptoms begin during the first few weeks of life and may persist until the age of 18 months, becoming more severe during episodes of upper respiratory tract infections or while crying, but subsiding in sleep.

Acute bronchitis

Acute bronchitis often follows a viral upper respiratory tract infection; there is always a cough, which may be accompanied by wheezing. There is no fever or difficulty with feeding. The respiratory rate is normal and the symptoms resolve within a week. The only signs, which are not always present continuously, are wheezes. Since bronchitis is usually due to a virus, antibiotics are indicated only if secondary bacterial infection is suspected.

Acute bronchiolitis

Acute bronchiolitis is an acute infection that occurs in winter epidemics in infants aged under 1 year. For the first few days there may be only a rasping cough but deterioration may occur within a few hours, causing a raised respiratory rate, indrawing of the intercostal spaces, cyanosis, drowsiness and apparent enlargement of the liver. The respiratory syncytial virus is found in over 70% of cases. During epidemics the disease may be recognized at an early stage, but at the beginning of epidemics the condition may be recognized only when the infant is moribund. Signs in the chest vary at different stages of the illness and there may be no adventitious sounds. The chest radiograph may appear normal even in severely ill infants. In units with immunofluorescence techniques for diagnosing respiratory syncytial virus results are available the same day, treatment can be planned, and cross-infection can be avoided. Oxygen is the most important aspect of treatment and is efficiently given by a nasal cannula with a special low flow regulator. Most infants need intragastric tube feeding or intravenous fluids for a few days. Where a viral cause can be confirmed immediately, antibiotics can be avoided but they should not be withheld from severely ill infants, as there is a possibility of additional bacterial infection. A few infants develop progressive respiratory distress and intermittent positive pressure ventilation may have to be considered.

The infant is discharged from hospital when feeding is normal. The cough may persist for 6 weeks, but if there is no improvement after 3 weeks, a sweat test should be performed to exclude cystic fibrosis.

Bronchopneumonia and segmental pneumonia

Pneumonia is acute inflammation of the lung alveoli. In bronchopneumonia the infection is spread throughout the bronchial tree whereas in segmental pneumonia it is confined to the

Box 21.4 **Upper limits for normal respiratory and heart rate per minute at rest related to age**

Age	Respiratory rate	Heart rate
<2 months	60	160
2–11 months	40	160
12–24 months	35	150

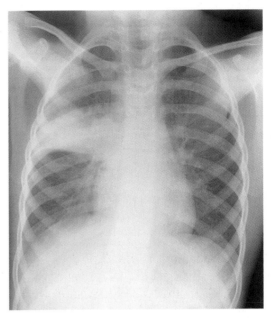

Figure 21.10 Chest radiograph showing pneumonia in the right lung.

alveoli in one segment or lobe. A raised respiratory rate at rest or indrawing of the intercostal spaces distinguishes pneumonia from bronchitis. The upper limit for a normal respiratory rate is related to age (Box 21.4). Cough, fever and flaring of the alae nasi are usually present and there may be reduced breath sounds over the affected area as well as crepitations. A chest radiograph, which is needed for every child with suspected pneumonia, may show extensive changes when there are no localizing signs in the chest (Figure 21.10). The radiograph may show an opacity confined to a single segment or lobe, but there may be bilateral patchy changes. Bacterial cultures of throat swabs and blood should be performed before treatment is started. Ideally, nasopharyngeal secretions should be studied virologically and virus antibody titres of serum collected in the acute and convalescent phases should be measured.

Children with pneumonia are best treated in hospital, as they may need oxygen treatment. Antibiotics should be prescribed for all cases of pneumonia, although a viral cause may be discovered later. If the child is not vomiting and not severely ill, oral amoxicillin or erythromycin is given. Cefotaxime is given intravenously if the symptoms are severe, and erythromycin is added when failure to improve promptly suggests infection with mycoplasma or chlamydia. Antibiotic treatment can be modified when the results of bacterial cultures are available. Intravenous fluids may be needed.

The chest radiograph of a child with segmental or lobar pneumonia should be repeated after 1 month.

Recurrent respiratory infections

Although all doctors concerned with children are familiar with the catarrhal child, the exact pathology of the condition is unknown and it is called by many names – postnasal discharge, perennial rhinitis or recurrent bronchitis. These children have an increased incidence of colds, tonsillitis and acute otitis media. Recurrent episodes of symptoms such as fever, nasal discharge and cough are most common during the second half of the first year of life, the years at playgroup or nursery school, and the first 2 years at primary school. Recurrent viral or bacterial infections contracted from siblings or fellow pupils may be important, but the considerable differences between the immune response of children in the same family suggest the possibility of a temporary immunological defect. During the winter several of these individual episodes may appear to join together to form an illness which lasts several months. On direct questioning, the mother will have observed a definite remission, if only for a few days between distinct episodes. If there are no remissions, especially if there has been vomiting, whooping cough should be considered (see below).

Various treatments including nasal drops and oral preparations of antihistamines are given with little effect. A chest radiograph should be performed to exclude persistent segmental or lobar collapse (Figure 21.11). A sweat test should be carried out to exclude cystic fibrosis and plasma immunoglobulin studies should be conducted to exclude rare syndromes. A Mantoux should be considered, although interpretation may be difficult if the child has received BCG (see page 104).

Recurrent bronchitis

Two separate episodes of acute bronchitis may occur in a normal child in a year. If attacks are more frequent at any age, bronchial asthma should be considered (Box 21.5). Viruses cause the majority of attacks of bronchitis and will precipitate most attacks of bronchial asthma. Some paediatricians have reverted recently to the older terms recurrent or wheezy bronchitis, as most children with these features become free of symptoms by the age of 5. Although the pathological processes and prognosis may differ between recurrent bronchitis and bronchial asthma, there is no clinical or laboratory method of distinguishing between them and treatment is the same.

After an episode of severe symptoms during an infection with respiratory syncytial virus (bronchiolitis), many children have recurrent episodes of cough and wheezing during the subsequent 4 years. It is not known whether the respiratory syncytial virus predisposes the child to recurrent respiratory symptoms or whether the child has a predisposition to produce severe symptoms with viral respiratory infections. If there is a persistent or recurrent cough, a chest radiograph should be performed to exclude persistent segmental or lobar collapse. A Mantoux test for tuberculosis and a sweat test to exclude cystic fibrosis should be performed and plasma concentrations of immunoglobulins and IgG subclasses should be measured to exclude transient or permanent immune deficiencies.

The management of recurrent bronchitis or bronchial asthma is the same. For infants with mild symptoms an oral bronchodilator, for example salbutamol, can be given at the beginning of an episode and continued for a week. If this is not effective, a bronchodilator can be given by a small spacer device with a face mask or by air pump and nebulizer (Figures 21.12 & 21.13). Infants with severe or frequent episodes can be given an inhaled steroid as a prophylactic drug for 6 weeks and the course can be extended to 6 months if there is an improvement in symptoms.

Prophylactic drugs can also be given with a small spacer device or by an air pump and nebulizer. If infants are receiving both a bronchodilator and a prophylactic drug, the dose of bronchodilator should be given just before the prophylactic drug.

Whooping cough

Young infants receive no protective immunity to whooping cough from their mothers and have the highest incidence of complications. Immunization is directed at increasing herd immunity

---

Box 21.5 **Causes of recurrent cough and wheezing**

- Recurrent bronchitis
- Asthma

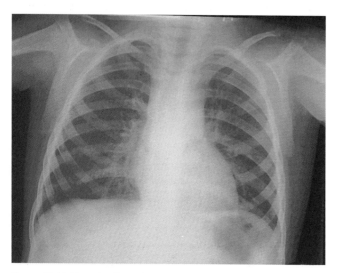

Figure 21.11 Normal radiograph.

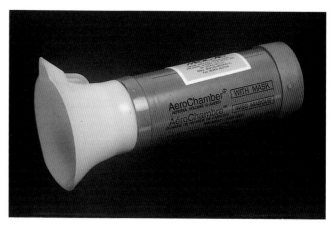

Figure 21.12 Small spacer device with a face mask.

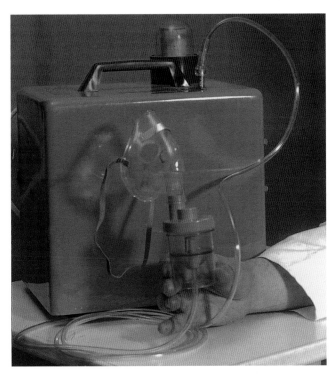

Figure 21.13 Air pump and nebulizer.

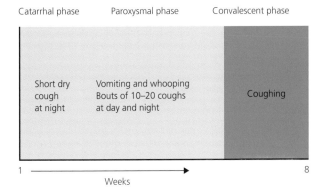

Catarrhal phase	Paroxysmal phase	Convalescent phase
Short dry cough at night	Vomiting and whooping Bouts of 10–20 coughs at day and night	Coughing

1 —————————————→ 8

Weeks

Figure 21.14 Phases of whooping cough.

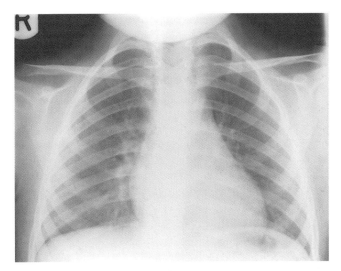

Figure 21.15 Normal chest radiograph.

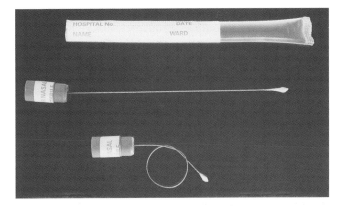

Figure 21.16 Pernasal swab for culture of *B. pertussis*.

and reducing the exposure of infants to older children who have the disease.

Diagnosis

Whooping cough is difficult to diagnose during the first 7–14 days of the illness (catarrhal phase), when there is a short dry cough at night (Figure 21.14). Later, bouts of 10–20 short dry coughs occur day and night; each is on the same high note or rises in pitch. A long attack of coughing is followed by a sharp indrawing of breath, which may produce the crowing sound or whoop. Some children, especially babies, with *Bordetella pertussis* infection never develop the whoop. Feeding with crumbly food often provokes a coughing spasm, which may culminate in vomiting. Afterwards there is a short period when the child can be fed again without provoking coughing. In uncomplicated cases there are no abnormal respiratory signs (Figure 21.15).

The most important differential diagnosis in infants is bronchiolitis; this is usually due to the respiratory syncytial virus, which produces epidemics of winter cough in infants under 1 year. For the first few days there may be only bouts of vibratory rasping cough, which never produce a whoop. Later, wheezes or crackles are heard in the chest and the infant either deteriorates or improves rapidly within a few days. Older siblings infected with the virus may have a milder illness. Other viruses may cause acute bronchitis with coughing, but there are seldom more than two coughs at a time.

A properly taken pernasal swab plated promptly on a specific medium should reveal *B. pertussis* in most patients during the first few weeks of the illness (Figure 21.16). A blood lymphocyte count of 10×10^9/L or more with normal erythrocyte sedimentation rate suggests whooping cough. The diagnosis may be confirmed in infants with a clinical diagnosis late in the illness by blood antibody tests to *B. pertussis*.

Management

If the diagnosis is suspected in the catarrhal phase (usually because a sibling has had recognizable whooping cough) a 10-day course of erythromycin may be given to the child and to other children in the home. Parents must be warned that an antibiotic may shorten the course of the disease only in the early stages and is unlikely to affect established illness. Vomiting can be treated by giving soft, not crumbly, food or small amounts of fluid hourly.

No medicine reliably reduces the cough. In severe cases parents can be taught to give physiotherapy, which may help to clear secretions, especially before the infant goes to sleep. An attack may be stopped by a gentle slap on the back.

The threshold for admission to hospital should be lower for children aged under 6 months. Convulsions and cyanosis during coughing attacks are absolute indications for admission to an isolation cubicle. Parents often become exhausted by sleep loss and arranging for different members of the family to sleep with the child will give them a respite. The cough usually lasts for 8–12 weeks and may recur when the child has any new viral respiratory infection during the subsequent year. If the child is generally ill or the cough has not improved after 6 weeks, a chest radiograph should be performed to exclude bronchopneumonia or lobar collapse, which need treatment with physiotherapy and antibiotics. Long-term effects on the lung, such as bronchiectasis, are rare in developed countries.

The infant will not be infective for other children after about 4 weeks from the beginning of the illness or about 2 days after erythromycin is started. The incubation period is about 7 days and contacts who have no symptoms 2 weeks after exposure have usually escaped infection.

Tuberculosis

Tuberculosis (TB) is a major problem in developing countries and is increasing in prevalence in inner city areas. Children usually contract the infection by inhaling airborne droplets containing *Mycobacterium tuberculosis* from an adult. Most children with TB are identified because they are contacts of an affected adult. The bacteria enter the lungs, tonsils or small intestine and cause enlargement of the adjacent lymph nodes or spread to the blood. The infection may be carried to the meninges, bones, joints, kidneys and pericardium. The main symptoms are prolonged fever (more than 10 days), chronic cough, malaise and weight loss. The signs in the lungs may include pneumonia or a pleural effusion.

The diagnosis is confirmed by a chest radiograph and an intradermal injection of tuberculin purified protein derivative (PPD), which is called the Mantoux test. The injection site is checked for swelling 2 days later. Gastric washings may be cultured. Treatment consists of a combination of drugs for 6 months. It is essential that all the doses are given to avoid the emergence of strains of *M. tuberculosis* which are resistant to standard treatment.

Immunization against TB is given in the neonatal period with an attenuated vaccine (BCG) to infants at high risk. These families are from areas of high prevalence of TB. High risk includes a close relative or contact of the family who is receiving treatment for TB or has had treatment for TB in the previous 10 years. Those with parents or grandparents born in countries with a high prevalence of TB also receive the vaccine. The vaccine produces a papule that enlarges over a few weeks and may ulcerate. It heals after about 8 weeks leaving a scar.

Further reading

Advanced Life Support Group. (2005) *Advanced Paediatric Life Support*, 4th edn. Blackwell Publishing, Oxford.

Block CL. (2006) Searching for the Holy Grail of acute otitis media. *Archives of Disease in Childhood* 91: 959–61.

CHAPTER 22

Fever in the Older Infant

OVERVIEW

- Fever may be present in the prodromal period of any of the infectious diseases of childhood but specific symptoms and signs should be sought to diagnose a more serious cause
- A urinary tract infection should be considered if there are no signs of another disease. Confirmation is by collecting a clean-catch urine sample, testing it with a dipstix for white cells and nitrites and sending it to the laboratory for microscopy and culture

Examining an ill child

Infants should be allowed to adopt whatever position they like (usually on their mother's knee) where they can be observed. The history taken must contain enough detail to provide a differential diagnosis before the physical examination begins.

The alertness, colour of the lips and respiratory rate should be observed before approaching the infant. A systematic examination may prove impossible in a protesting infant, so the most relevant system should be examined first. If the infant objects to being fully undressed, only the part being examined need be exposed. The examiner needs warm hands and should talk to the infant continuously to soothe him or her. Patience and gentleness at this stage are often rewarded by the infant accepting a full examination without protest.

The baby's abdomen is best examined as the infant lies on their mother's knees during a feed. Abdominal breathing is normal and the edge of the liver is easily palpable. Even the newborn will show abdominal tenderness by grimacing or crying. Rectal examination may be performed with the little finger.

Instruments such as auriscopes and stethoscopes should be shown to the infant first and rested on their forearm so that they can see what they are (Figure 22.1). The auriscope must be used gently and the speculum not pushed too far into the external meatus. When the pinna is pulled gently outwards and downwards, the tympanic membrane can be seen with the tip of the speculum in the outer end of the meatus (Figure 22.2).

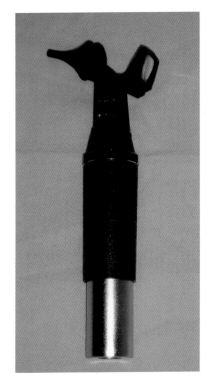

Figure 22.1 Auriscope.

Examination of the throat, which is the most disliked procedure, should be left until last (Figure 22.3). It should never be performed in an infant with stridor unless the examiner has the facilities to intubate the infant immediately.

The infant should be examined again no longer than 24 hours later and the initiative for this review should not be left to the parents, who may not appreciate the danger of features that have developed.

The normal oral or rectal temperature is about 37.5°C (99.5°F) and the normal axillary (skin) temperature 37.0°C (98.4°F). If the temperature is 0.5°C above these levels, the infant has a fever. In the prodromal period of any infectious disease of childhood, fever may be the only symptom.

Specific causes

Tonsillitis. There may be small areas of pus on the tonsils or the throat may be generally red. The presence of pus does not

ABC of the First Year, Sixth edition. By B. Valman and R. Thomas. © 2009 Blackwell Publishing, ISBN: 978-1-4051-8037-5.

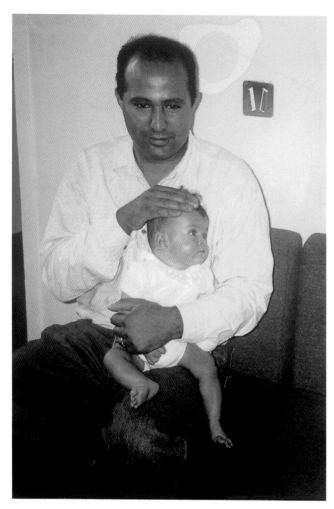

Figure 22.2 Ear examination.

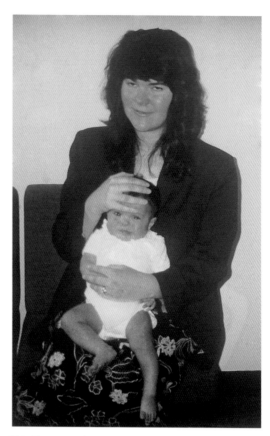

Figure 22.3 Throat examination.

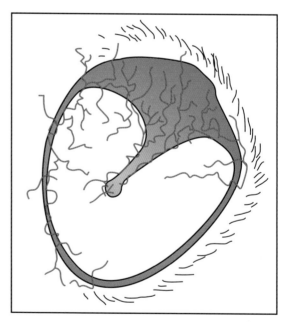

Figure 22.4 Acute otitis media.

help to distinguish between bacterial infection due to group A streptococcus (*Streptococcus pyogenes*) and a viral infection. Petechiae on the soft palate usually indicate a viral infection. A throat swab should be taken and a 10-day course of oral penicillin given (see page 98).

Acute otitis media. An early sign is an increase in the size of the vessels of the upper posterior part of the drum (Figure 22.4). Later the drum becomes dull pink or red and in severe cases there is bulging. Ear drums can be examined efficiently only if the auriscope has a magnifying lens. It is important to look for swelling or tenderness over the mastoids. The first choice of drugs is oral amoxycillin or erythromycin. If these are not effective, amoxycillin with clavulanic acid or cefalexin is given. The drum should be examined again after 2 days and if there is no improvement the antibiotic should be changed.

Septicaemia. There are no specific signs. The infant appears extremely ill. In meningococcal septicaemia there may be a generalized purpuric rash (Figure 22.5). Intravenous or intramuscular penicillin (300 mg) should be given immediately and the infant admitted, with the doctor taking the child to hospital personally if necessary. An infant with meningococcal septicaemia may die within a few hours of the onset of symptoms.

Meningitis. Irritability, drowsiness and vomiting are common. A convulsion accompanied by fever may be the first sign. Neck stiffness is rare and raised anterior fontanelle tension is a late sign. Unusual drowsiness is a sinister symptom.

Roseola. Although fever may be present in the prodromal period of any infectious disease of childhood, pronounced fever is a

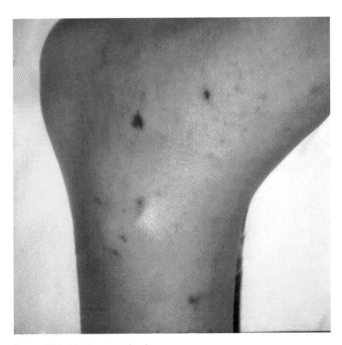

Figure 22.5 Meningococcal rash.

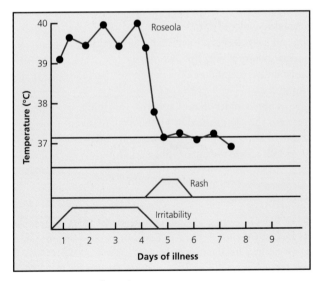

Figure 22.6 Features of roseola.

the diagnosis or exclusion of a urinary tract infection. A baby less than 3 months of age or a child with abdominal pain should be seen by a paediatric specialist within a few hours. The child may have to be admitted because an accurate diagnosis and prompt treatment with intravenous antibiotics may be needed. If the child is more than 3 months and has no features of an acute illness a course of trimethoprim is started and the treatment can be changed if necessary the following day when the results of antibiotic sensitivity tests are received.

A clean-catch urine specimen is the ideal. Only social cleanliness and dryness are required. An alternative is a special urine pad which is removed as soon as it has become wet. If these techniques are not effective, a bag urine specimen should be obtained while the infant is held upright and the specimen transferred from the bag as soon as it is passed. A negative result from a bag urine specimen is reliable, but a positive result should be confirmed by a clean-catch specimen, by suprapubic puncture or, rarely, by a catheter specimen. If suprapubic aspiration is needed, the infant should be referred to hospital for day care or inpatient investigation.

The specimen of urine should ideally be collected in a sterile container, cooled immediately to 4°C, and examined in the laboratory within 2 hours. Before the specimen is sent to the laboratory it is tested with a dipstix for nitrites which indicate whether an infection is probable or unlikely. The method and time of collection must be stated on the pathology request to enable the microbiologist to give an accurate opinion. An alternative is to refrigerate the specimen at 4°C in the main compartment of a domestic refrigerator for, at most, 48 hours before examination. The temperature of the general practice refrigerator should be checked regularly. Another possibility is to transport the urine in 1.8% boric acid, but the correct amount of urine must be added to the bottle to ensure the correct concentration of boric acid.

Infants aged under 6 months who have responded to antibiotics within 48 hours should have an ultrasound examination of the renal tract within 6 weeks. Infants who fail to respond or who have recurrent urinary infections may need further investigations including isotope renal scanning and cystourethrography. Isotope renal scanning detects scars, ultrasound examination shows obstructive lesions, and cystourethrography detects vesicoureteric reflux and should be performed under the protection of a suitable antibiotic (Figure 22.7).

Urine cultures are performed at times of fever or recurrence of symptoms. Infants older than 6 months who have had a single urinary tract infection with no fever or abdominal pain need no imaging investigations. If the infection recurs, investigations with an initial ultrasound examination are indicated.

notorious feature of roseola infantum, which is caused by human herpesvirus 6 or 7 (Figure 22.6). It usually occurs between 6 months and 3 years. The temperature usually reaches 39–40°C and remains at this level for about 3 days. The temperature falls as discrete minute pink macules appear on the trunk; these may spread to the limbs within a few hours. The infant appears less ill than might be expected from the height of the fever. The suboccipital, cervical and postauricular lymph nodes are often enlarged and the blood picture frequently shows neutropenia.

Urinary tract infection in children often presents simply with fever (Box 22.1). It is essential that a carefully taken specimen of urine is tested for nitrites with a dipstix and sent to the laboratory promptly. The presence or absence of proteinuria is of no value in

Pneumonia. A raised respiratory rate at rest and fever may be the only signs of pneumonia and a chest radiograph may be necessary

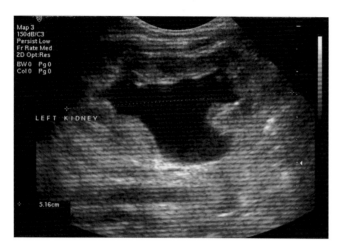

Figure 22.7 Ultrasound scan of kidney: dilated renal pelvis.

to show consolidation. The upper limit for the normal respiratory rate is 60/min for infants less than 2 months of age and 40/min between 2 and 12 months. Movements of the alae nasi and indrawing of the chest wall between the ribs are confirmatory signs.

Osteomyelitis or septic arthritis may present with fever. In the early stages the only helpful sign may be the infant's reluctance to move a limb and radiographs are often normal. Later there is redness, swelling and tenderness at the site of the osteomyelitis, which usually affects the maxilla, long bones or vertebrae in infants. Early blood culture and radioisotope bone scans are helpful in the diagnosis.

Malaria. If within the previous 2 years the child has been in an area where malaria is endemic, blood films should be examined immediately for malarial parasites (Figure 22.8). The parasites are most numerous during fever but may be found at any time.

Kawasaki disease. Persistent fever lasting more than 3 days should prompt the consideration of Kawasaki disease. Features include conjunctivitis, cracked lips, red throat, cervical lymphadenopathy, blotchy rash, oedema of the hands and feet, and reddening of the palms and soles. In the second week there may be peeling of the skin of the fingertips and toes. Prompt admission for intravenous gammaglobulin reduces the risk of coronary artery aneurysms.

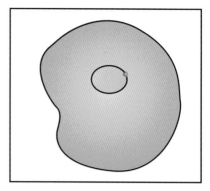

Figure 22.8 Malarial parasite in red cell.

Pyrexia of undetermined origin

If children simply have fever, ideally they should be observed for 6 hours in an ambulatory care unit or admitted to a cubicle on a children's ward for observation. Usually these children will have a full blood count, CRP or ESR, urine microscopy and culture and sometimes blood culture and CSF examination.

Infants older than 3 months with no symptoms or signs apart from pyrexia may be considered for management at home provided that they have all the following positive features:
- normal response to a smile
- continuously alert and interested in surroundings
- normal colour of skin, lips and tongue
- moist mucus membranes
- strong cry.

If the infant is older than 3 months and fulfils the criteria for home care, the carer should be given an appointment for a further assessment at a specific time and place and guidance as to when and how to seek care in the intervening period.

Further reading

National Institute for Health and Clinical Excellence. (2007) *Feverish illness in young children.* NICE clinical guideline 47. www.nice.org.uk/CG47
National Institute for Health and Clinical Excellence. (2007) *Urinary tract infection in children.* NICE clinical guideline 54. www.nice.org.uk/CG54

CHAPTER 23

Convulsions in the Older Infant

OVERVIEW

- Febrile convulsions are common and there is often a family history. Most children who have febrile convulsions do not develop epilepsy. Parents are very frightened when they witness a convulsion in their child for the first time and need reassurance that the child is not going to die
- Epilepsy can present at any age, including the newborn period. An electroencephalogram and brain imaging should be arranged if convulsions are unilateral, focal or prolonged

In infants between the ages of 1 month and 1 year convulsions are usually associated with fever. If there is no fever, epilepsy should be considered.

Fits can be divided into generalized or partial seizures. Generalized seizures include tonic-clonic and myoclonic fits. Partial seizures include focal and temporal lobe fits. During some episodes partial seizures may be followed by generalized seizures.

Generalized tonic-clonic fits are the most common type (Boxes 23.1 & 23.2). The child may appear irritable or show other unusual behaviour for a few minutes before an attack. Sudden loss of consciousness occurs during the tonic phase, which lasts 20–30 seconds and is accompanied by temporary cessation of respiratory movements and central cyanosis. The clonic phase follows and there are jerky movements of the limbs and face (Figure 23.1).

Box 23.1 **Features of a tonic–clonic convulsion**

Tonic
- Cry
- Loss of consciousness
- Rigidity
- Apnoea

Clonic
- Repetitive limb movement (rate can be counted)

Sleep

ABC of the First Year, Sixth edition. By B. Valman and R. Thomas. © 2009 Blackwell Publishing, ISBN: 978-1-4051-8037-5.

Box 23.2 **Dangers**

- Inhalation of vomit
- Hypoxaemia

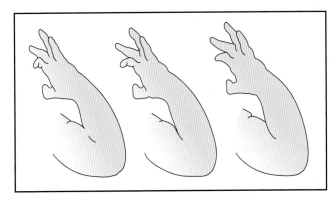

Figure 23.1 Repeated similar movements indicate a convulsion.

The movements gradually stop and the child may sleep for a few minutes before waking confused and irritable.

Although a typical tonic-clonic attack is easily recognized, other forms of fits may be difficult to diagnose from the mother's history. Infantile spasms may begin with momentary episodes of loss of tone, which can occur in bouts and be followed by fits in which the head may suddenly drop forward or the whole infant may move momentarily like a frog. Recurrent episodes with similar features, whether they are changes in the level of consciousness or involuntary movements, should raise the possibility of fits.

Differential diagnosis

Convulsions must be differentiated from blue breath-holding attacks, which usually begin at 9–18 months. Immediately after a frustrating or painful experience, some infants cry vigorously and suddenly hold their breath, become cyanosed, and in the most severe cases lose consciousness. Rarely, their limbs become rigid and there may be a few clonic movements lasting a few seconds. Respiratory movements begin again and infants gain consciousness immediately. The attacks diminish with age with no specific treatment. Parents may be helped to manage these extremely frightening episodes by being told that the child will not die and that they should handle each attack consistently by putting the child on their side and waiting for the symptoms to settle.

Rigors may occur in any acute febrile illness, particularly urinary tract infections, but there is no loss of consciousness.

Febrile convulsions

A febrile convulsion is a fit occurring in a child aged from 6 months to 5 years, precipitated by fever arising from infection outside the nervous system in a child who is otherwise neurologically normal.

Convulsions with fever include any convulsion in a child of any age with fever of any cause. Among children who have convulsions with fever are those with pyogenic or viral meningitis, encephalitis or cerebral palsy with intercurrent infections. Children who have a prolonged fit lasting more than 30 minutes or who have not completely recovered within 1 hour should be suspected of having one of these conditions.

Most of the fits that occur between the ages of 6 months and 5 years are simple febrile convulsions and have an excellent prognosis (Box 23.3).

By arbitrary definition, in simple febrile convulsions the fit lasts less than 20 minutes, there are no focal features, and the child is aged between 6 months and 5 years and has been developing normally prior to the convulsion.

Often fever is recognized only when a convulsion has already occurred. Febrile convulsions are usually of the tonic–clonic type. The objective of emergency treatment is the prevention of a prolonged fit (lasting over 30 minutes), which may be followed by permanent brain damage, epilepsy and developmental delay.

An electroencephalogram (EEG) is not a guide to diagnosis, treatment or prognosis.

Emergency treatment

A child who has fever should have all his or her clothes removed and should be covered with a sheet only. They should be nursed on their side or prone with their head to one side because vomiting with aspiration is a constant hazard (Figure 23.2).

Buccal midazolam (0.3 mg/kg per dose up to 2.5 mg as a single dose) produces an effective blood concentration of anticonvulsant within 10 minutes and can be easily administered by parents or carers. Rectal diazepam (0.5 mg/kg) is also very effective and can be administered using a convenient preparation resembling a toothpaste tube (Stesolid); however, this route of administration has become less acceptable in recent years. Early admission to

hospital or transfer to the intensive care unit should be considered if a second dose of anticonvulsant is needed.

Some children who have had a first febrile convulsion should be admitted to hospital to exclude meningitis and to educate the parents, as many fear that their child is dying during the fit. Physical examination at this stage usually does not show a cause for the fever, but a specimen of urine should be examined in the laboratory to exclude infection and a blood glucose test should be performed. Blood should be taken for blood culture and plasma glucose and calcium estimations. Most of these children have a generalized viral infection with viraemia. A febrile convulsion may occur in roseola at the onset and 3 days later the rash appears. Occasionally, acute otitis media is present, in which case an antibiotic is indicated, but most children with febrile convulsions do not need an antibiotic. A purpuric rash suggests meningococcal septicaemia and the need for ceftriaxone or penicillin to be given immediately either intravenously or intramuscularly (see page 106).

Lumbar puncture

A lumbar puncture should be considered if the child is under 18 months old or any of the following are present:

- signs of meningism such as neck stiffness
- drowsiness, irritability or systemic illness
- complex convulsion that contains any feature that does not conform with the definitions of a simple convulsion.

Ideally, the decision should be taken by an experienced doctor, who may decide on clinical grounds that lumbar puncture is unnecessary even in a younger child, but when in doubt the investigation should be performed. If the convulsion is prolonged or has unusual features, a CT brain scan should be performed before the lumbar puncture. The doctor deciding not to undertake a lumbar puncture should review the patient personally within a few hours. Children less than 2 years of age may have meningitis with no neck stiffness or other specific signs.

A child who has had severe vomiting or is in coma must be examined by an experienced doctor and have a CT brain scan before lumbar puncture because of the risk of coning.

Management of fever

There is no evidence that antipyretic treatment influences the recurrence of febrile convulsions, but fever should be treated to promote the comfort of the child and to prevent dehydration.

Box 23.3 **Simple febrile convulsions**

All the following:

- < 20 minutes
- No focal features
- 6 months to 5 years of age
- No developmental or neurological abnormalities
- Not repeated in the same episode
- Complete recovery within 1 hour

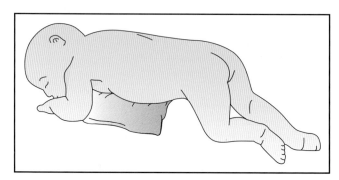

Figure 23.2 Position should be on the side or prone with the head to one side.

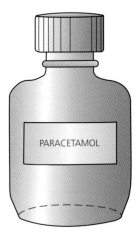

Figure 23.3 Paracetamol is the preferred antipyretic.

The child's clothes should be taken off and he or she should be covered with a sheet only. Paracetamol is the preferred antipyretic and adequate fluid should be given (Figure 23.3).

Failure to respond to paracetamol is an indication to give ibuprofen.

Anticonvulsant drugs

Buccal midazolam or rectal diazepam should be used as soon as possible after the onset of the convulsion. The parents should be advised not to give it if the convulsion has stopped. The only indication for long-term anticonvulsant prophylaxis after febrile convulsions is a prolonged initial convulsion or frequent recurrences. There is no evidence that the prophylactic use of anticonvulsant drugs in the minority of children who later develop epilepsy would have prevented it.

Immunization

As routine immunization is given to children 2–4 months old, this schedule is usually completed before febrile convulsions occur. Babies having convulsions with fever aged under 6 months should be assessed by a paediatrician. Children who have febrile convulsions before immunization against diphtheria, pertussis, pneumococcus, meningococcus and tetanus because the immunization has been delayed, should be immunized after their parents have been instructed about the management of fever and the use of rectal diazepam or buccal midazolam (Figure 23.4).

Measles, mumps and rubella immunization should be given as usual to children who have had febrile convulsions, with advice about the management of fever to the parents. Buccal midazolam or rectal diazepam should be made available for use should a convulsion occur.

Prognosis

Unless there is clinical doubt about the child's current developmental or neurological state, parents should be told that the prognosis for development is excellent. The risk of subsequent epilepsy after a single febrile convulsion with no complex features is about 1%. With each additional complex feature the risk rises to 13% in those children with two or more complex features (Box 23.4). Only about 1% of children with febrile convulsions are in this group.

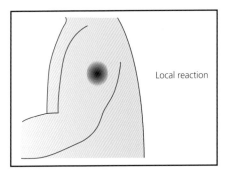

Figure 23.4 Immunization may be followed by a febrile convulsion.

Box 23.4 **Features of complex febrile convulsions**

- Lasting > 30 minutes
- Focal
- More than one on the same day
- Developmental or neurological abnormalities

The risk of having further febrile convulsions is about 30%. This risk increases in younger infants and is about 50% in infants aged under 1 year at the time of their first convulsion. A history of febrile convulsions in a first-degree relative is also associated with a risk of recurrence of about 50%. A complex convulsion or a family history of epilepsy is probably associated with an increase in the risk of further febrile convulsions.

Information for parents

Information for parents should include:

- an explanation of the nature of febrile convulsions, including information about the prevalence and prognosis
- instructions about the management of fever, the management of a convulsion, and the use of buccal midazolam
- reassurance about the benign nature of febrile convulsions.

Both verbal and written advice should be given (see below).

Advice to parents: Febrile convulsions

Your child has had a febrile convulsion. We know it was a very frightening experience for you. You may have thought that your child was dead or dying, as many parents think that when they first see a febrile convulsion. Febrile convulsions are not as serious as they appear.

What is a febrile convulsion?
It is an attack brought on by fever in a child aged between 6 months and 5 years.

What is a convulsion?
A convulsion is an attack in which the child becomes unconscious and usually stiff, with jerking of the arms and legs. It is caused by unusual electrical activity of the brain. The words convulsion, fit and seizure have the same meaning.

(Continued)

Continued

What shall I do if my child has another convulsion?
Lay him on his side, with his head on the same level or slightly lower than the body. Note the time. Do not try to force anything into his mouth. Do not slap or shake the child.
The hospital may give you medicine to insert into your child's mouth or for rubbing into the gums. This is called buccal midazolam. This treatment should stop the convulsion within 10 minutes. If it does not, take your child to the hospital. You may need to dial 999 to obtain an ambulance. Let your doctor know what has happened.
About 1 child in 30 will have had a febrile convulsion by the age of 5 years.

Is it epilepsy?
No. The word epilepsy is applied to fits without fever, usually in older children and adults.

Do febrile convulsions lead to epilepsy?
Rarely; 99 out of 100 children with febrile convulsions never have convulsions after they reach school age, and never have fits without fever.

Do febrile convulsions cause permanent brain damage?
Almost never. Very rarely, a child who has a very prolonged febrile convulsion lasting half an hour or more may suffer permanent damage from it.

What starts febrile convulsions?
Any illness that causes a high temperature, usually a cold or other virus infection.

Will it happen again?
Three out of 10 children who have a febrile convulsion will have another one. The risk of having another febrile convulsion falls rapidly after the age of 3 years.

Does the child suffer discomfort or pain during a convulsion?
No. The child is unconscious and unaware of what is happening.

What shall I do if my child has fever?
You can take the child's temperature by placing the bulb of the thermometer under his armpit for 3 minutes with his arm held against his side. Give plenty of fluids to drink. Give children's paracetamol or ibuprofen to reduce the temperature.
If the child seems ill or has ear ache or sore throat, let your doctor see him or her in case any other treatment, such as an antibiotic, is needed. Antibiotics are not necessary for most children with fever due to virus infections.

Is regular treatment with tablets or medicine necessary?
Usually not. The doctor will explain to you if your child needs regular medicine.

Adapted from a pamphlet produced by the British Paediatric Association

Basic life support in the community

Basic life support (BLS) should be given immediately whenever an infant stops breathing, even if no specialized equipment is available. It may be life saving.

Box 23.5 **Sequence of basic life support**

Call for help
Check environment is safe
Assess condition

Airway

Breathing

Circulation

Assessment of condition
The level of consciousness of the infant should be quickly assessed by gentle pressure on the shoulders or limbs together with a verbal command. Even young infants may open their eyes or move in response to sound if they are not unconscious. Young infants should not be shaken as this may result in brain haemorrhage from trauma caused by the mobile brain hitting the inside of the skull. If the infant is not responsive, then the ABC of basic life support should be followed (Box 23.5).

Airway
The rescuer can assess whether the infant is breathing by placing their face closely above the infant's face in order to look, listen and feel for breathing and chest movement. If the infant is not breathing, the head of the infant should be maintained in the neutral position (head in line with body) by gentle pressure with one of the rescuer's hands on the forehead and chin lift or jaw thrust under the angles of the mandible with the other hand (Figure 23.5a). Flexion or overextension of the neck of an infant may cause obstruction of the upper airway by the tongue blocking the pharynx. Attempts to improve an obstructed airway with the rescuer's finger are not recommended and may be dangerous.

Breathing
The rescuer should give five exhaled breaths, each lasting approximately 1 second into the infant's mouth or mouth and nose. The chest of the infant should be seen to expand with each breath or else the airway is not clear and airway-opening manoeuvres should be repeated.

Circulation
After five initial breaths, the pulse should be assessed by palpation of the brachial artery in the medial aspect of the antecubital fossa or femoral artery in the groin (Figure 23.5b). The carotid artery is difficult to palpate in infants because the neck is often short and fat. If the pulse is absent or <60 beats/min as assessed over 10 seconds, then external cardiac compressions should be commenced.

External cardiac compression (Figure 23.5c,d)
Cardiac compressions should be applied with the infant lying flat on the back on a firm surface. There are two methods of compressions in small infants.
1 Hands encircling the thorax with the thumbs compressing the sternum one fingerbreadth below an imaginary line drawn between the nipples. This method is only possible in very small infants and is difficult for a lone rescuer to perform along with mouth to mouth with or without nose breaths.

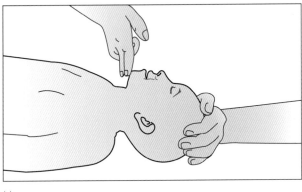

(a)

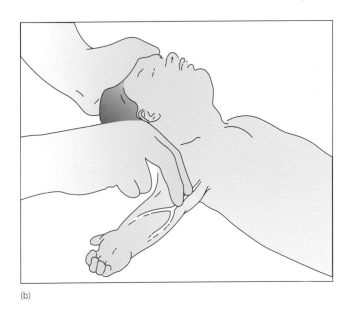

(b)

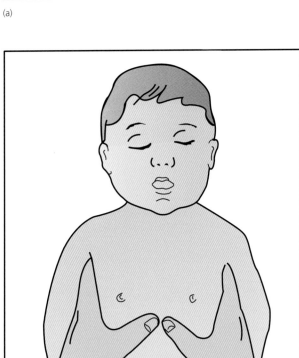

(c)

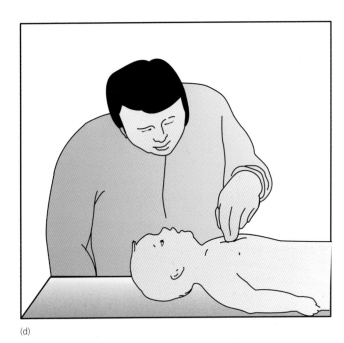

(d)

Figure 23.5 (a) Chin lift in an infant. (b) Feeling for the brachial pulse. (c) External cardiac compression. (d) External cardiac compression.

2 Two-finger technique with the ball (not tips) of two fingers compressing the chest, with the fingers again placed one fingerbreadth below the imaginary line between the nipples.

Whichever method is used, the chest should be compressed by about one-third depth in order to propel blood to the coronary arteries.

Continue CPR

Cardiopulmonary resuscitation (CPR) should be continued with a ratio of 15 chest compressions to two breaths for approximately 1 minute before reassessment. The compression rate is 100/min. It is not necessary to simulate the heart rate of a normally breathing infant and, indeed, it may not be possible to do so in an effective manner. The rescuer should continue CPR until the emergency services arrive and take over resuscitation, or if no help has arrived within a few minutes, the infant should be carried quickly to where help can be summoned.

Further reading

Mackway-Jones K, Molyneux E, Phillips B, Wieteska S, eds. (2005) *Advanced Paediatric Life Support*, 4th edn. Blackwell Publishing, Oxford.

Sadleir LG, Scheffer IE. (2007) Febrile seizures. *British Medical Journal* 334: 307–11.

CHAPTER 24

Crying Babies and Sleep Problems

OVERVIEW

- Babies who cry excessively have difficulty in sleeping
- The problems are common in infants less than 3 months of age. Hunger, thirst, feeding problems and acute illness are the common causes in this group
- After 3 months loneliness, separation from the mother and social changes are the most common reasons for excessive crying
- Prevention is by a bedtime ritual which may consist of a bath and a story
- A behaviour modification plan may resolve persistent symptoms

Apart from the subtle method of eye-to-eye communication, babies have no other way of signalling their needs to their carers than by crying (Figure 24.1). Babies who are quiet or 'good' may be abnormal or ill. As crying is a non-specific call for help, obvious needs should be investigated. In most cases no remediable cause is found and the problem may resolve spontaneously when infants are about 3 months old.

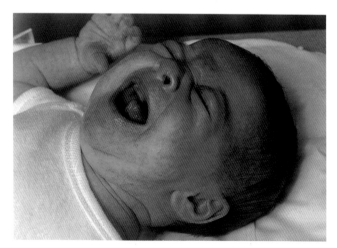

Figure 24.1 Crying signals needs.

ABC of the First Year, Sixth edition. By B. Valman and R. Thomas. © 2009 Blackwell Publishing, ISBN: 978-1-4051-8037-5.

By then, however, parents may have become exhausted from lack of sleep and marital discord may follow while the infant remains fresh. As well as suggesting any appropriate management, the family doctor should encourage parents to take one or two evenings off together each week to visit friends or go to a film. Parents often worry that the infant is suffering from lack of sleep and wrongly ascribe poor appetite or frequent colds to this cause.

Sound spectrography has confirmed the clinical impression that cries of cerebral irritability, pain and hunger are different in quality, but this method is not available to most clinicians. During the first month infants do not shed tears when they cry and even after the age of about 6 months many infants cry at night without shedding tears.

The doctor needs to take a full history, including details of the pattern of crying, when the problem began, and measures taken to resolve it. It should be possible to determine whether the infant has always needed little sleep or whether he or she has developed a habit of crying in order to get into his or her parents' comfortable bed. The doctor should also explore the reason why the parents have sought advice at this stage. The mother should be asked about any change in the house, where the infant sleeps, and who looks after him or her during the day. Illnesses in the child or family, and marital and social backgrounds also need considering. A physical examination usually shows no abnormality, but occasionally there may be signs of acute otitis media.

Difficulty in getting to sleep may be avoided by starting a bedtime ritual in infancy. A warm bath followed by being wrapped in particular blankets may later be followed by the mother or father reading from a book or singing nursery rhymes before the light is turned out (Figures 24.2 & 24.3). A soft cuddly toy can lie next to the infant from shortly after birth, and seeing this familiar toy again may help to induce sleep.

It is recommended that the infant should sleep in a cot in the parents' room for the first 6 months of life. The parents should be told that during the night babies often open their eyes and move their limbs and heads. They should be asked to resist getting up to see their baby, as the noise of getting out of bed may wake them and they may then remain awake. Babies who do wake may be pacified with a drink and may then fall asleep.

Parents whose young children sleep a great deal during the day can discourage them from doing this by taking them out shopping or giving them other diversions, and they may then sleep well at night.

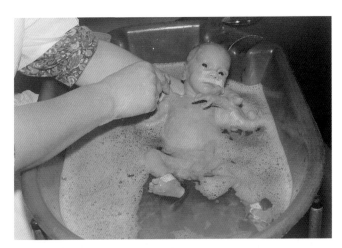

Figure 24.2 A bath is a bedtime ritual.

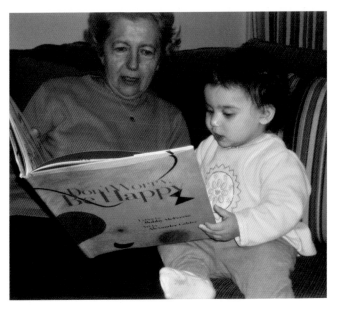

Figure 24.3 Grandmother reading from a book.

Sleep disturbance is a common reaction to the trauma of admission to hospital or moving house, and taking the child into the parents' room for a few weeks may help to reassure the infant that they have not been abandoned.

If the infant is prepared to go to sleep at a certain time but the parents would like to advance it by an hour, they may be able to put him or her to bed 5 minutes earlier each night until the planned bedtime is achieved.

Hunger and thirst

Babies often cry and become restless just before a feed is due and in the early weeks of life the infant may demand to be fed 3-hourly or even 2-hourly. This is perfectly normal. Preterm infants need particularly high milk intakes for 'catch-up' growth and they may become less hungry when they have reached their final centiles for weight.

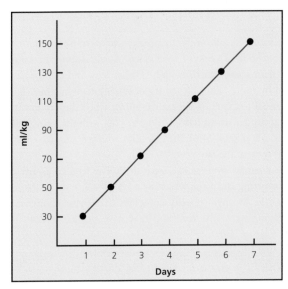

Figure 24.4 Milk intake increases with age.

The volumes of bottled milk recommended are only average amounts and many infants will therefore need more to prevent excessive hunger. Regular weighing and use of a growth chart to plot the results are the only ways of ensuring that the infant is obtaining the correct amount of feeds (Figure 24.4). Feeding at regular intervals is apt to cause crying in many babies and demand feeding is preferable. Some infants scream when they approach the breast and the help of an experienced midwife is needed to overcome this problem.

The age at which infants sleep through the night and do not require a night feed varies greatly. It usually occurs when infants weigh about 5 kg and parents may be worried because their neighbour's child of a similar age has already omitted the night feed. Similar competition between mothers over which baby first manages three meals a day may also lead to inadequate feeding, followed by crying.

It is impossible to determine the difference between a cry due to hunger and a cry due to thirst. The only way of solving this problem is to offer infants water twice daily. This can easily be given mid-morning or mid-afternoon.

Even newborn infants cry to obtain physical contact and the crying stops as soon as they are picked up (Figure 24.5). It does not spoil babies to pick them up when they want contact. Once they are a few weeks old infants begin to have periods of waking and some will not tolerate being left in a pram or cot by themselves. A harness that allows them to remain in contact with their mother's body will often satisfy these infants. Alternatively, a canvas chair can be used even as early as 1 month and can be placed in a safe position in the kitchen or wherever the mother is working.

If babies do not stop crying when held, walking with them, rocking them, or taking them for a car ride may stop the crying. Wrapping infants in a blanket and putting them firmly into a carrycot or a very small cot may also provide contact, although by an impersonal method.

Non-nutritive sucking stops crying, provided babies are not hungry. Putting a dummy (pacifier) into the mouth of a crying baby who is not hungry may be effective as a temporary measure.

Three months' colic and feeding problems

Three months' colic is the name given to a syndrome that usually begins at about 2 weeks of age and has usually stopped by 4 months. The infant screams, draws up his or her legs, and cannot be comforted by milk, being picked up or having their napkin changed. This usually occurs in the early evening, when the mother is busy getting supper ready, has less time to play with the baby, and may be anxious (Figure 24.6). Breastfeeding mothers may have less milk at that time of the day.

Some babies swallow excessive air during feeding as a result of milk spurting from the breast or a very small hole in the teat of the bottle. Mothers usually complain that these infants gulp at the beginning of the feed and they have particular difficulty in

bringing up the wind. This problem does not occur in societies where babies are held on the mothers' backs for most of the day. The infant's abdomen is pressed against the mother's back and the infant is kept upright, which is the best position for releasing excessive gastric air.

If the milk spurts from the breast, the first 25 mL or so should be expressed manually and given to the infant later if necessary. If the baby is fed by bottle, the size of the hole in the bottle teat should be checked and made larger with a hot needle if necessary. Infants can be winded most easily by putting them prone with their head higher than their feet, but they must be observed constantly while in this position.

Teeth and teething

Although mothers consider that the eruption of the first tooth is a milestone in development, the age at which this occurs is of no practical importance. The first teeth to appear, at 6–12 months, are the lower incisors.

From the age of a few weeks infants normally put their fingers, and later anything else that comes to hand, into their mouths and mothers often wrongly ascribe this to teething.

Teething produces only teeth. It does not, contrary to common belief, cause convulsions, bronchitis or napkin rash. Some mothers insist their infants are particularly irritable when they are teething, but it is important to examine the infant to exclude disease such as otitis media or meningitis before accepting the mother's explanation.

Dummies temporarily affect the growth of the mouth but there are no objections to using them. They should not be dipped in honey. Severe dental caries also follows the use of 'comforters' or 'dinky-feeders', which are filled with fluid containing sugar.

Tetracycline or its derivatives should never be given to children less than 8 years of age, as permanent brownish-yellow staining of the teeth may occur (Figure 24.7).

Other causes

Illness. If the infant starts crying persistently, especially if he or she has not cried like this before, disease should be suspected. Acute otitis

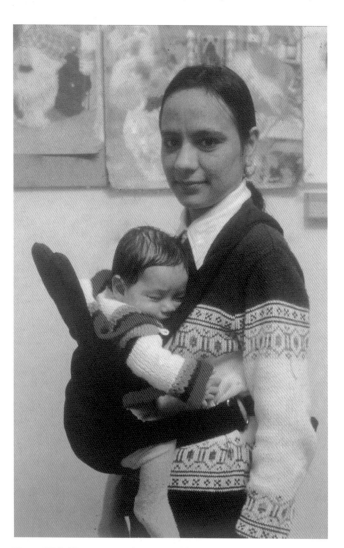

Figure 24.5 Close contact often stops crying.

Figure 24.6 Evening colic begins about 5 pm.

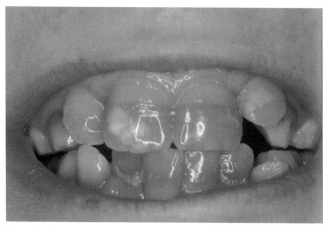

Figure 24.7 Severe discoloration due to tetracycline.

media often causes persistent crying at night, but meningitis or a urinary tract infection may have no specific signs. An intussusception is an invagination of a proximal part of the gut into a more distal portion and may result in partial or complete intestinal obstruction. The infant has sudden attacks of screaming and pallor that last for a few minutes and recur every 10–20 minutes. Between attacks the infant appears normal. Bloodstained mucus may be passed rectally. The abdomen is tender only during attacks, but often there is a mass over the course of the colon. If intussusception is suspected the infant should be admitted to hospital (see page 59).

Mechanical problems. Babies do not seem distressed when their napkins are wet or soiled, though some cry when they are being undressed or changed. An open safety pin is an extremely rare cause of crying.

Fatigue. When young infants have been on a long journey or have been stimulated more than usual by playing with relatives, they may become irritable and not keen to sleep.

Failure of mother–infant adjustment. Crying may be a sign of this failure, which may be related to the character of the infant as much as the response of the mother. The crying may represent the difficulties of each adjusting to the other. If an infant has been crying persistently for several weeks the possibility of severe depression in the mother should be considered. This depression could be the cause or the result of the crying. The mother is exhausted by lack of sleep and particularly liable to injure her infant, and both mother and infant may need to be admitted to hospital for diagnosis and management (Figure 24.8).

For most infants none of the above reasons for crying are present. The parents need reassuring strongly after examination that their infant is healthy and that the problem will resolve spontaneously. Sedation of the infant with chloral hydrate for a week during a difficult period may enable the mother to regain some of her strength.

Special problems after the age of 3 months

Loneliness is probably the commonest cause of crying after the age of 3 months. While they are awake during the day some infants will not tolerate being left alone but are happy if they are left in the room where the mother is working (Figure 24.9). These infants are extremely interested in their surroundings and need the stimulation of things going on around them. Similarly, infants need to be propped up when out in their prams and when they begin to reach out they need simple toys to play with (Figure 24.10).

Separation from the mother during admission to hospital or when parents go on holiday by themselves may be followed by

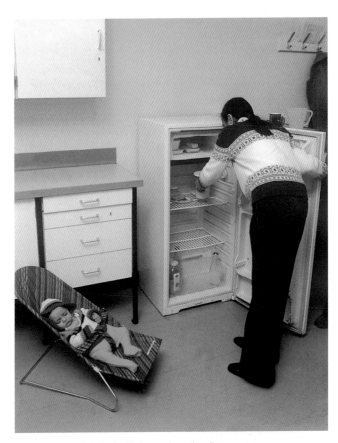

Figure 24.9 A chair in the kitchen reduces loneliness.

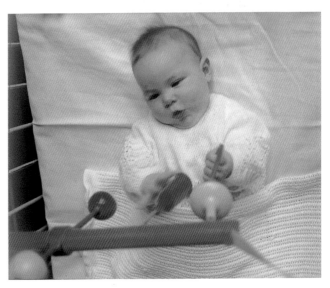

Figure 24.10 Playing with toys suspended across the cot.

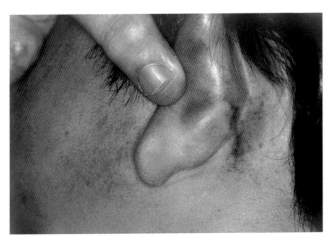

Figure 24.8 Non-accidental injury behind the ear.

bouts of crying. An infant can relate to only two or three adults at a time and frequent changes in carer may be associated with crying.

After about 5 months infants may cry when a stranger approaches them or when they sleep in a different room. They may wake suddenly and appear terrified, which might be due to a nightmare, although there is no method of proving this.

Infants who do not sleep after 3 months

During the first few weeks of life some babies sleep almost continuously for the 24 hours whereas others sleep for only about 12 hours. Many mothers consider that a newborn baby should sleep continuously and do not realise that babies take an interest in what is going on around them. Infants who need little sleep may wake regularly at 2 or 4 am and remain awake for 2 or 3 hours. Some are settled by a drink, but others cry persistently and the mother may take the infant into her own bed before they go to sleep. This should be avoided as the mother may roll on the baby and cause an injury. Some infants wake in a similar way but are then content to remain awake looking at mobiles above their cots or playing with toys left in the cot.

Behaviour modification and drugs

When infants wake frequently during the night and cry persistently, a plan of action is needed. If there is an obvious cause, such as acute illness or recent admission to hospital, the problem may resolve itself within a few weeks, and at first there need be no change in management. If there is no obvious cause, the parents are asked to keep a record of the infant's sleep pattern for 2 weeks (see Figure 24.11). This helps to determine where the main problem lies and can be used as a comparison with treatment.

Both parents are seen at the next visit; both need to accept that they must be firm and follow the plan exactly. Behaviour modification is the only method that produces long-term improvement, but it can be combined with drugs initially if the mother is at breaking point.

Behaviour modification separates the mother from the child gradually or abruptly, depending on the parents' and doctor's philosophy. The slow method starts with the mother giving a drink and staying with the child for decreasing lengths of time. In the next stage no drink is given. Then she speaks to the child through the

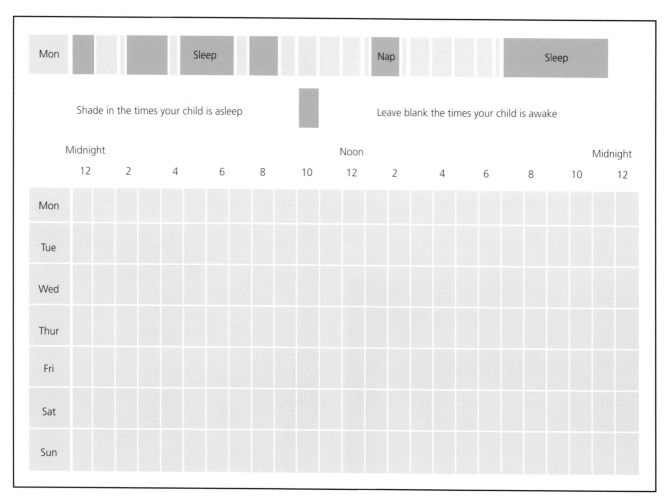

Figure 24.11 Record of sleep pattern.

Day	Time to bed	Time to sleep	First problem	What did you do?	Second problem	What did you do?	Time woke up in morning
Mon							
Tue							
Web							
Thur							
Fri							
Sat							
Sun							

Figure 24.12 Record of action by parents.

Day	At first episode	If your child is still crying		
		Second episode	Third episode	Subsequent episodes
1	5	10	15	15
2	10	15	20	20
3	15	20	25	25
4	20	25	30	30
5	25	30	35	35

Figure 24.13 Number of minutes to wait before going into your child briefly.

closed door and, finally, does not go to the child at all. The abrupt method consists of letting the child cry it out; he or she stops after 3 or 4 nights. There are an infinite number of variations between these extremes and the temperament of the parents, child and doctor will determine what is acceptable (Figure 24.12).

Another approach is to increase the waiting time before going to the infant (Figure 24.13). In severe cases a written programme of several small changes can be given to the mother and she can be seen again by the health visitor or family doctor after each step has been achieved. The mother will need to be reassured that the infant will not develop a hernia from crying or vomit or choke, and neighbours may be pacified by being told that the child will soon be cured.

Many sleep problems can be resolved without drugs, but some mothers are so exhausted by loss of sleep that they cannot manage a programme of behaviour modification unless the infant receives some preliminary sedation. The most satisfactory drug for this age group is chloral hydrate 30 mg/kg body weight given 1 hour before going to bed. The full dose is given for 2 weeks, followed by a half dose for a week; the drug is then given on alternate nights for a week. The objective is to change the pattern of sleeping. A behaviour modification plan is needed during the third and subsequent weeks.

CHAPTER 25

Non-accidental Injury

This section has been restricted to physical abuse, as sexual abuse is rare in infants less than a year of age. Non-accidental injury inflicted by adults on children is often hard to detect. Symptoms that are difficult to explain may be the result of

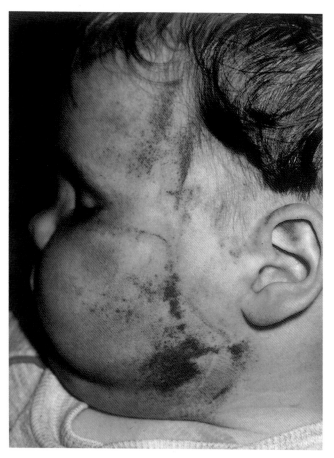

Figure 25.1 Non-accidental injury.

inflicted injury. In the UK as many as 100 children a year may die from non-accidental injuries. Non-accidental injury should be suspected, especially in a child aged under 3, whenever: (a) there has been a delay between the accident occurring and the parents seeking medical help; (b) the explanation of the injury is inadequate, discrepant or too plausible; (c) the child or sibling has a history of non-accidental or suspicious injury; (d) there is evidence of earlier injury; (e) the child has often been brought to the family doctor or accident department for little apparent reason; (f) the parents show disturbed behaviour or unusual reactions to the child's injuries or have a history of psychiatric illness; (g) the child shows obvious neglect or failure to thrive.

Typical initial injuries are: (a) burns, abrasions or small bruises on the face; (b) injuries to the mouth or torn frenulum of the tongue; (c) bruises caused by shaking or rough handling, including finger-shaped bruises; (d) subconjunctival or retinal haemorrhages. If the doctor suspects non-accidental injury, the child should be undressed completely and examined fully, with all signs of injury noted (Figure 25.1). If the doctor's suspicions are not allayed, he or she should ensure the immediate examination of the child by a consultant paediatrician. The family doctor should, if possible, not mention any suspicions to the parents, as they may refuse to allow this examination and it may impair his or her relationship with them.

Children with genuinely accidental injuries will occasionally be admitted unnecessarily, but this should not deter any doctor from admitting a child when there is reasonable doubt about the cause of an injury.

Further reading

Crawford M, Ghulam S, Herbison J, Hobbs C, Mok J, Mott A, Price J, eds. (2006) *Child Protection Companion*. Royal College of Paediatrics and Child Health, London.

ABC of the First Year, Sixth edition. By B. Valman and R. Thomas. © 2009 Blackwell Publishing, ISBN: 978-1-4051-8037-5.

Chapter 26

Selected Drugs

Newborn

Intestinal absorption is variable and regurgitation of antibiotics common, so the intravenous route should usually be used initially. Intramuscular injections are given into the upper lateral aspect of the thigh. Schemes for rotation of sites are essential to prevent local necrosis and to avoid further injections being given into a relatively avascular area. Drugs are usually given intramuscularly or orally every 8 hours and intravenously by slow bolus injection every 12 hours. In preterm infants an adjustment of dose and frequency of administration may be needed and specific texts should be consulted. Table 26.1 applies to the first month.

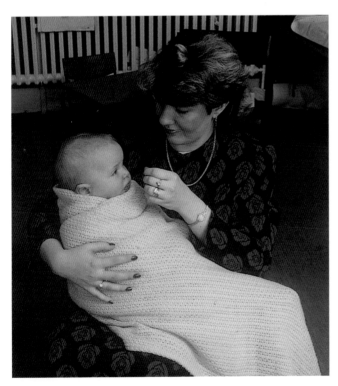

Figure 26.1 Wrapping the infant may prevent spillage of medicine.

ABC of the First Year, Sixth edition. By B. Valman and R. Thomas. © 2009 Blackwell Publishing, ISBN: 978-1-4051-8037-5.

Table 26.1 Selected drugs in the newborn.

Amoxicillin oral	
Under 7 days	62.5–125 mg twice daily
1 week–1 year	62.5–125 mg 3 times daily
Ampicillin oral	
Under 7 days	62.5 mg–125 mg twice daily
7–21 days	62.5–125 mg 3 times daily
21 days–1 year	62.5–125 mg 4 times daily
Ceftazidime iv	
Under 7 days	25–50 mg/kg once daily
7–21 days	25–50 mg/kg twice daily
21 days–1 year	25–50 mg/kg 3 times daily
Chloral hydrate oral	
Newborn	30–50 mg/kg per dose
Diazepam	
iv 1 day–1 year	300–400 micrograms/kg per dose
Rectal newborn	1.25–2.5 mg per dose
Flucloxacillin oral	
Under 7 days	25 mg/kg twice daily
7–21 days	25 mg/kg 3 times daily
21–28 days	25 mg/kg 4 times daily
Gentamicin iv	2.5 mg/kg 12-hourly. Blood concentration
Term infant–1 month	must be checked
Miconazole gel oral	
Newborn	1 mL twice daily
Naloxone im	10–20 micrograms/kg per dose
Nystatin oral	
Newborn	100 000 units/dose (after feeds)
Paraldehyde rectal	
Newborn	0.4 mL/kg per dose
Benzylpenicillin iv	
Under 7 days	25–50 mg/kg twice daily
7–28 days	25–50 mg 3 times daily
Phenobarbitone iv or oral	
Newborn	20 mg/kg iv once only followed by 2.5–5 mg/kg per dose once daily orally
Phenytoin iv or oral	
Newborn	20 mg/kg per dose slowly once iv followed by 2–4 mg/kg per dose twice daily orally
Sodium ironedetate oral	
Newborn	1 mL twice daily
Trimethoprim oral	
Newborn	3 mg/kg as single dose then 1–2 mg/kg twice daily

Table 26.2 Selected drugs in older infants.

Amoxiycillin oral	62.5–125 mg 3 times daily
Ampicillin oral	62.5–125 mg 4 times daily
Betamethasone iv or im	1 mg per dose = 30 mg hydrocortisone
Cefalexin oral	125 mg twice daily
Cefotaxime iv or im	50 mg/kg 2–4 times daily
Chloral hydrate oral	30–50 mg/kg per dose
Chlorpheniramine im or iv	250 micrograms/kg per dose
Diazepam iv	300–400 micrograms/kg slowly intravenously
rectal	5 mg/dose
Erythromycin oral	125–250 mg 4 times daily
Flucloxacillin oral	62.5–125 mg 4 times daily
Gentamicin iv or im	2.5 mg/kg 3 times daily
Hydrocortisone	25 mg per dose intramuscularly or intravenously
Ibuprofen	5–10 mg/kg 4 times daily
Nystatin oral	100 000 units per dose (after feeds)
Paracetamol oral	10–20 mg/kg 4 times daily
rectal	20–30 mg/kg 4 times daily
Paraldehyde rectal	0.15 mL/kg per dose
Benzylpenicillin im or iv	25–50 mg/kg 4 times daily
Phenoxymethylpenicillin oral	12.5 mg/kg 4 times daily
Trimethoprim	4 mg/kg twice daily. Single daily prophylactic dose 2 mg/kg

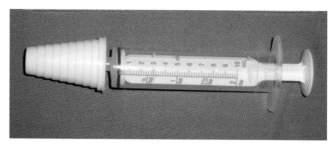

Figure 26.2 Special medicine syringes (which have no needles) can be used to measure and give small volumes accurately.

preparations, particularly the penicillins, have an unpleasant taste and the medicine should not be mixed with food as the infant may then hate both. Syrup, which is a sucrose solution that forms the base of most elixirs, may cause dental caries if it is given regularly for a long time. If only one adult is present to give the medicine, wrapping the infant securely in a blanket may prevent spillage (Figure 26.1). Special medicine syringes (which have no needles) can be used to measure and give small volumes accurately (Figure 26.2). The doses in Table 26.2 apply to infants between 1 month and 1 year.

Further reading

BNF for Children 2007. BMJ Publishing Group, London. www.bnfc.org
Paediatric drug information line 0151 252 5837 info@dial.org.uk
The Contact a Family Directory 0808 808 3555 www.cafamily.org.uk
This charity provides advice, information and support to parents of all disabled children and enables parents to get in touch with other families with a similar condition.

Older infants

Infants treated at home and most of those in hospital need oral drugs three times a day. The drugs should be given before feeds and the infant need not be woken specially for them. Some

Index